T0100146

THE INTERNATIONAL JOURNAL OF ETHICAL LEADERSHIP

Special Volume: 2
Inamori International
Thesis Prize in Military Ethics
2021 | 2022

English—Español—Français

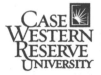

CASE WESTERN RESERVE UNIVERSITY

INAMORI INTERNATIONAL
CENTER FOR ETHICS
AND EXCELLENCE

The International Journal of Ethical Leadership
Case Western Reserve University
Editor-in-Chief: Shannon E. French, Inamori Professor in Ethics and
    Director, Inamori International Center for Ethics and Excellence
Executive Editor: Michael Scharf, Dean of the School of Law, John
    Deaver Drinko-Baker & Hostetler Professor of Law, and Director,
    Frederick K. Cox International Law Center
Senior Executive Editor: Beth Trecasa, Associate Director,
    Inamori International Center for Ethics and Excellence
Copyeditor: Thea Ledendecker

For additional information, please contact inamoricenter@case.edu
or visit case.edu/inamori

Contents

Message from the Editors

Shannon E. French
Inamori Professor in Ethics and Director,
and
Beth Trecasa
Associate Director,
Inamori International Center for Ethics and Excellence
Case Western Reserve University

Dear *IJEL* Readers,

The Inamori International Center for Ethics and Excellence at Case Western Reserve University awards an annual prize for the best thesis in military ethics to promote active involvement in the study and application of military ethics. This interdisciplinary field focuses on a wide range of issues including Just War Theory (JWT; also referred to as the Just War Tradition); the conduct of war (*jus in bello*); the pursuit of a just peace (*jus ad pacem*); the Law of Armed Conflict (LOAC); International Humanitarian Law (IHL); and other related topics such as the development of new military technologies (example: autonomous weapons systems); what societies owe to those who serve in their militaries; moral injury and dehumanization; and human rights in the context of armed conflict.

The prize winning theses featured in this volume help illustrate the wide range of issues tackled by those who study military ethics. In 2021, first place went to Laura Graham for, "Malum In Se: Starvation Crimes in International Law." Second place went to Nathan Riehl for "The Virtuous (Human) Soldier: A MacIntyrian Approach to Moral Education in the US Army." Graham's work examines the horrific and wide scale harms caused by the use of intentional starvation of civilians as a weapon of war and explains why it must be recognized and prosecuted as a war crime (and the challenges of doing so). Riehl's thesis makes the case for professional military education (PME) in ethics to be based on a nuanced philosophical understanding of virtue ethics. Our 2022 winner, Sara Gaines, wrote on "Artificial Intelligence as Clinician: An Argument for Ethical Use of Future Technology in a Medical Setting." This topic cuts across three key areas of applied ethics: bioethics, ethics of emerging technology, and military ethics—specifically, military medical ethics. Gaines explores the promise, risks, and limits of the potential use of computerized systems to aid human medics in some of the most ethically challenging and emotionally/psychologically fraught situations, such as battlefield triage.

We encourage applications for the Inamori thesis prize in military ethics from any non-European students, either military or civilian, in a graduate or professional-level program (including law or medical students, etc.) studying for their degree at any accredited college or university or military service academy or war college (or similar). We have purposely focused the prize in this way to complement a similar thesis award available to Europeans offered by the esteemed Euro-ISME (International Society for Military Ethics, European Chapter) organization. Israeli scholars are now also eligible for the Euro-ISME prize. Due to our partnership with Euro-ISME, winners of the Inamori thesis prize have the opportunity to present their work at the prestigious annual Euro-ISME conference, which is a unique global gathering of top scholars in the field. Our 2022 winner was able to present her work in person at the 2022 Euro-ISME annual conference, while our 2021 winners presented theirs virtually, due to the pandemic.

In an effort to foster global discussion of pressing issues in military ethics and improve the general accessibility of the field, the Inamori Center is publishing the winning theses, in print and online, in multiple languages. This special volume of *The International Journal of Ethical Leadership* includes our 2021 and 2022 winners in English, Spanish, and French. We are grateful to our multilingual partners who make this kind of publication possible. Translation is a unique skill, and it is exceptionally complicated work when it involves precise legal and ethical arguments and terminology. Without our talented translators and proofreaders, we would never be able to have such a truly global conversation.

Sincerely,

Shannon and Beth

Malum in se
Starvation Crimes in International Law

Laura K. Graham

Starvation has been used as a method of warfare since time immemorial. Yet, despite developments in the laws of armed conflict (LOAC) over the past 150 years aimed at the prohibition of starvation of civilians during war, the use of starvation as a method of warfare persists. This is because belligerents have two lawful means with which to use starvation: (1) siege warfare and (2) blockades aimed at cutting off supplies to the enemy. In this paper, I will argue that even where belligerents employ starvation warfare under the color of international humanitarian law (IHL), such tactics are never morally justified and should be absolutely prohibited because starvation is *malum in se*—i.e., starvation is an innately immoral act, regardless of whether IHL strictly prohibits it. This is so because when used as a weapon of war, starvation violates *jus in bello* principles.

In Part I, I examine the historical IHL and international criminal law (ICL) developments of prohibitions—or rather permissions—on the use of starvation during armed conflicts beginning with the Lieber Code of 1863 and ending with the 2019 amendment to the Rome Statute prohibiting starvation in non-international armed conflicts and defining it as war crime. In Part II, I present my arguments that starvation is *malum in se* because it violates the *jus in bello* principles of distinction, proportionality, necessity, and superfluous injury. In Part III, I present two case studies—one historical and one contemporary—where starvation has been used as a weapon of war. I first present the Nazi Hunger Plan to highlight the immoral position of using starvation against the enemy. Then, I present the contemporary case of Yemen's civil war where thirteen million people are at risk of starving or dying from starvation-related disease because of the Saudi-led Coalition's attacks on agriculture, water, and objects indispensable to survival (OIS). These case studies demonstrate that even under the color of law, using hunger as a weapon of war is *malum in se* and should be absolutely prohibited and punished under international law. Finally, I conclude by advocating for stricter prohibitions on starvation under international law with some strategies for pursuing this aim.

Part I. Historical Developments on Prohibitions of Starvation as a Method of Warfare

The laws of war—*jus in bello* or international humanitarian law—govern the conduct of parties to an armed conflict and what military tactics are permissible in a just war.[1] Among the core humanitarian rules of warfare in the 19th and 20th centuries were the principles of military necessity and proportionality—the idea that parties to an armed conflict may undertake an attack when it is actually necessary to accomplish a legitimate military purpose, but it must be balanced with the principle of proportionality to minimize civilian harm.[2] Oppenheim's treatise, *International Law*, describes the first and second principles of the laws of war—necessity and humanity—as a contradiction that must be reconciled.[3] International humanitarian law, in the form of regulations and conventions, thus developed to reconcile the necessities of war with the principle of humanity.

Prohibitions on *unnecessary* use of starvation as a method of warfare can be traced back to the 1863 Lieber Code, which acknowledges that starvation of the enemy is permissible to hasten capitulation, but that civilian casualties must meet the IHL principles of necessity and proportionality—i.e. civilian deaths must be necessary and proportionate to a legitimate military objective, such as bringing an end to war.[4] Developed for the US Union Army during the Civil War, the Lieber Code provides:

> War is not carried on by arms alone. It is lawful to starve the
> hostile belligerent, armed or unarmed, so that it leads to the

---

1. International humanitarian law is generally regarded as having developed after Henry Durant witnessed the 1859 Battle of Solferino and established the Red Cross movement. The Lieber Code is considered the first example of a codification of the laws of war. However, the laws of war and international humanitarian law, though often used interchangeably, are actually distinct: Geneva law, deriving from the early Geneva Conventions, represent customs of humanitarian principles, whereas Hague law, deriving from the 1899 and 1907 Hague Peace Conferences, represent the conventional rules of the conduct of war. Most legal scholars no longer treat the Hague and Geneva laws as distinct. *See* Amanda Alexander, "A Short History of International Humanitarian Law," *European J. of Int'l L.* 26 (2015): 109, 112–116.

2. *See, e.g.,* Judith Gardam, *Necessity, Proportionality and the Use of Force by States* (Cambridge University Press 2004 e-book) 28–30 (explaining that necessity and proportionality had been part of just war theory since the Middle Ages); General Order No. 100 (April 24, 1863) Lieber Code, Instructions for the Government of Armies of the United States in the Field, Arts. 14–16, https://avalon.law.yale.edu/19th_century/lieber.asp#sec1 [hereinafter, Lieber Code].

3. *See, e.g.,* L. Oppenheim, *International Law: A Treatise*, edited by R. F. Roxburgh, 3rd ed. (1921), 84–85.

4. Lieber Code, *supra* note 3, at Arts. 17–18.

speedier subjection of the enemy. When a commander of a besieged place expels the noncombatants, in order to lessen the number of those who consume his stock of provisions, *it is lawful, though an extreme measure to drive them back, so as to hasten on the surrender.*[5]

Inherent in this code is the military necessity of using starvation in order to hasten capitulation. The use of a siege or blockade must be in pursuit of a legitimate military necessity—in other words, it would not be legitimate to use starvation to punish the enemy, exterminate a population, or pillage the enemy's territory for food and supplies to sustain a prolonged military campaign. Though the Lieber Code does not expressly mention proportionality, Article 18 could be interpreted as providing for proportionality insofar as the purpose of permitting siege warfare is to hasten surrender, therefore limiting the total number of casualties of war. What is lacking in the Lieber Code is the principle of humanity—that suffering of civilians in particular is impermissible and unjust. Thus, it would be too much to proclaim the Lieber Code as the first codification of the prohibition on starvation of civilians, but it could be viewed as the first step towards that end given the conditions of military necessity and proportionality implied in Articles 17–18.

Although no express prohibitions on the use of starvation of civilians existed in the 19th century, the 1899 Hague Convention could be construed to prevent starvation of civilians under the Martens Clause, which prohibits methods of warfare that would shock the public conscience.[6] The Martens Clause, articulated in the preamble of the 1899 Hague Convention II, provides:

> Until a more complete code of the laws of war is issued, the High Contracting Parties think it is right to declare that in cases not

---

5. Lieber Code, *supra* note 3, at Arts. 17–18 (emphasis added). The Lieber Code's permissions to drive combatants back into a besieged area in order to hasten the defeat of an enemy stands in stark contrast to the modern convention that, whenever possible, civilians and non-combatants must be allowed to leave a besieged area or humanitarian aid must be allowed through the siege for civilians. *See, e.g.,* Protocol Additional to the Geneva Conventions of 12 August 1949, and relating to the Protection of Victims of International Armed Conflicts (Protocol I), 8 June 1977, Arts. 54, 70.

6. The principle of humanity, sometimes referred to as the Martens clause, protects civilians from violations of IHL not expressly covered by treaties. It was introduced by Fyodor Fyodorovich Martens in the preamble of the 1899 Hague Convention. *See* ICRC, "Fundamental Principles of IHL," https://casebook.icrc.org/glossary/fundamental-principles-ihl.

included in the Regulations adopted by them, *populations and belligerents remain under the protection and empire of the principles of international law*, as they result from the usages established between civilized nations, *from the laws of humanity and the requirements of the public conscience.*[7]

The humanity principle is intended to act as a failsafe to prevent belligerents from engaging in anti-humanitarian warfare. It prohibits methods of warfare that are unnecessary for attaining a definite military advantage,[8] and is closely tied to the principle prohibiting weapons that cause superfluous injury.[9] Jean Pictet interpreted the principle of humanity to mean that "[N]on-combatants shall be spared as far as possible."[10] A broad interpretation is that even if a treaty or convention does not expressly prohibit an act or conduct of belligerents, that does not mean that the act or conduct is *ipso facto* permitted. Rather, such an act or conduct is subject to the principles of customary international law.[11] In the context of starvation, it can be argued that although no treaty or convention expressly prohibited starvation of civilians during World War II, the Martens humanity principle suggests that if the use of starvation as a method of warfare did not meet a legitimate military objective or was not proportionate, then it was not lawful under the customs of the time.

Further, the 1907 Hague Convention does not expressly mention starvation as a method of warfare, but does provide that siege warfare, which

---

7. Convention (II) with Respect to the Laws and Customs of War on Land and its annex: Regulations concerning the Laws and Customs of War on Land, The Hague, 29 July 1899, Preamble (emphasis added).

8. E. Kwakwa, *The International Law of Armed Conflict: Personal and Material Fields of Application* (Kluwer Academic, Dordrecht, 1992), 36.

9. Convention (II) with Respect to the Laws and Customs of War on Land and its annex: Regulations concerning the Laws and Customs of War on Land, The Hague, 29 July 1899, Preamble.

10. Jean Pictet, Development and Principles of International Humanitarian Law, Martinus Nijhoff and Henry Dunant Institute (Dordrecht/Geneva, 1985), 62.

11. Rupert Ticehurst, "The Martens Clause and the Laws of Armed Conflict," International Review of the Red Cross 317 (Apr. 30, 1997), https://casebook.icrc.org/glossary/fundamental-principles-ihl; But *see*, S. S. Lotus (Fr. v. Turk.), Judgment, 1927 P.C.I.J. Series A 16 No. 10 (Sept. 7), at 19 (In its dicta, the Court describes what has become known as the second Lotus Principle, which crudely suggests that anything not expressly prohibited by international law is permitted: "It does not, however, follow that international law prohibits a State from exercising jurisdiction in its own territory, in respect of any case which relates to acts which have taken place abroad and in which it cannot rely on some permissive rule of international law. Such a view would only be tenable if international law contained a general prohibition to States to extend the application of their laws and the jurisdiction of their courts to persons, property, and acts 'outside their territory'....").

has the effect of starving civilians and combatants alike, is permissible.[12] The 1907 Hague Convention reemphasized the humanity principle of the Martens Clause and the principle of necessity.[13] Thus, the 1907 Hague Convention could be interpreted as banning a military tactic like the Nazi Hunger Plan, which used starvation as a means of eliminating civilians, rather than bringing an end to war.

To that end, The International Military Tribunal at Nuremberg (IMT-N) declared that the 1907 Hague Convention's rules of war were customary international law in 1939:

> The rules of land warfare expressed in the [1907 Hague] Convention undoubtedly represented an advance over existing international law at the time of their adoption ...but by 1939 these rules ...were recognized by all civilized nations and were regarded as being declaratory of the laws and customs of war.[14]

However, despite the fact that the 1907 Hague Convention prohibits belligerents from causing unnecessary suffering and destruction of property,[15] the IMT-N did not charge Nazi perpetrators with the crime of starvation for the Hunger Plan. The IMT-N did, however, charge Field Marshal Wilhelm von Leeb for the Siege of Leningrad in the High Command trial. As the name suggests, the High Command trial was the prosecution of twelve Nazi high commanding officers for their alleged war crimes and crimes against peace during World War II; von Leeb's trial was for his role in the invasion of the Soviet Union during Operation Barbarossa. The IMT-N ultimately determined that although starvation by siege was egregious, it was nevertheless lawful:

> A belligerent commander may lawfully lay siege to a place controlled by the enemy and endeavor by a process of isolation to cause its surrender. The propriety of attempting to reduce it by starvation is not questioned. It is said that if the commander of a besieged place expels the noncombatants, in order to lessen

---

12. Articles 27 of the Hague Convention IV places prohibitions on belligerents to attack the sick and wounded during siege warfare, but not civilians specifically, and Article 28 prohibits pillaging of a besieged town or village. *See* Convention (IV) respecting the Laws and Customs of War on Land and its annex: Regulations concerning the Laws and Customs of War on Land. The Hague, 18 October 1907, Arts. 27–28 [hereinafter, Hague Convention IV].
13. *Id.* at Preamble.
14. International Military Tribunal at Nuremberg, reprinted in *AJIL* 41, 248–249 (1947).
15. Hague Convention IV, *supra* note 12, at Art. 23.

the number of those who consume his stock of provisions, *it is lawful, though an extreme measure, to drive them back so as to hasten surrender.*....Hence the cutting off every source of sustenance from without is deemed legitimate....*We might wish the law were otherwise, but we must administer it as we find it.* Consequently, we hold no criminality attached on this charge.[16]

Indeed, state practice would suggest that the major parties to World War II, with the exception of the Soviet Union, all believed that starvation for the purpose of causing the enemy to capitulate was a legitimate and legal method of warfare. For example, the US and UK used blockades of food supplies to Germany, German-Occupied Territory, and Japan; the US even named its blockade of Japanese harbors "Operation Starvation."[17] Thus, starvation caused by sieges and blockades during World War II was not *ipso facto* prohibited under international law. However, even though starvation was not strictly prohibited during World War II, that does not establish that the use of starvation during the war complied with the principles of military necessity, proportionality, distinction, or humanity.

The horrors of World War II led to two significant developments in international law: the 1948 Genocide Convention and the 1949 Geneva Convention for Treatment of Civilians—both of which expressly prohibit starvation of civilians.[18] The Genocide Convention prohibits "Deliberately inflicting on the group conditions of life calculated to bring about its physical destruction in whole or in part."[19] Starvation undoubtedly meets this criterion. More recently, the 1977 Additional Protocols to the Geneva Conventions provide detailed explanation of permissions and prohibitions on sieges, blockades, attacks on OIS, and humanitarian aid;[20] and the 1998 Rome Statute[21] and

---

16. Trials of War Criminals before the Nuernberg Military Tribunals Under Control Council Law No. 10, Nuernberg, October 1946–April 1949, Vol. XI, 563 (U.S. Government Printing Office, Washington, D.C., 1950) (emphasis added).

17. Alex De Waal, *Mass Starvation: The History and Future of Famine* (2018), 127–28.

18. Convention on the Prevention and Punishment of the Crime of Genocide, 9 December 1948, 78 U.N.T.S. 277, Art. II(c); Geneva Convention relative to the protection of civilian persons in time of war, Geneva 8 December 1949.

19. *Id.*

20. Protocol Additional to the Geneva Conventions of 12 August 1949 and Relating to the Protection of Victims of International Armed Conflicts (Protocol I), June 8, 1977, 1125 U.N.T.S. 3, at Art. 54(1) [hereinafter, Protocol I]; Protocol Additional to the Geneva Conventions of 12 August 1949 and relating to the Protection of Victims of Non-International Armed Conflict, June 8, 1977, 1125 U.N.T.S. 609, at Arts. 14, 69–70 [hereinafter, Protocol II].

21. Rome Statute of the International Criminal Court, Art. 8(2)(b)(xxv), 17 July 1998, UN

2019 Amendments criminalize starvation as a method of warfare during both international and non-international armed conflicts.[22] Specifically, Article 54 of Additional Protocol I and Article 14 of Additional Protocol II prohibit attacks on OIS and starvation of civilians, while Article 70 of Additional Protocol I requires uninhibited flow of humanitarian aid.[23] While starvation of civilians is strictly prohibited under Article 54, sieges and blockades are lawful exceptions to the prohibitions on starvation, so long as the attack complies with the principles of military necessity, distinction, and proportionality, and does not deprive civilians of adequate food or water, or force civilians to leave due to inadequate food or water.[24] Finally, the Rome Statute of the International Criminal Court (ICC) criminalizes starvation as a war crime when the perpetrator intends to cause starvation of civilians as a method of warfare, deprives civilians of OIS, or willfully impedes relief supplies.[25]

Although the law has evolved to enforce greater restrictions on methods of war that would lead to starvation, currently IHL, ICL, and customary international law stop short of an absolute ban on the use of starvation as a weapon of war. Hence, any change in the law must come as a result of progressive development. As I will lay out below, starvation should be absolutely banned under international law because it is *malum in se*. I will also apply the Doctrine of Double Effect (DDE) to some of the arguments that follow. DDE is a philosophical exercise that explains the permissibility of a harmful action, such as starvation of civilians, as a consequence of promoting some good intention, such as bringing an end to a protracted war. In order for an action to be morally permissible under DDE, four conditions must be satisfied:

1. The action must be morally good or morally indifferent;
2. The intention of the agent must be to bring about the good effect and not the bad one. If the agent could attain the good effect without the bad effect, then that is what is required;

Doc. A/CONF. 183/9, 2187 U.N.T.S. 9 [hereinafter, Rome Statute].

22. International Criminal Court Assembly of State Parties, Report of the Working Group on Amendments, Eighteenth session, 2–7 December 2019, 7–9, ICC-ASP/18/32 (Dec. 3, 2019), https://asp.icc-cpi.int/iccdocs/asp_docs/ASP18/ICC-ASP-18-32-ENG.pdf.
23. Protocol I, *supra* note 20, at arts. 54(1) & 70; Protocol II, *supra* note 20, at art. 14.
24. *Id.* at Additional Protocol I, art. 54(3).
25. Rome Statute, *supra* note 21, at art. 8(2)(b)(xxv)("Intentionally using starvation as a method of warfare by depriving civilians of objects indispensable to their survival, including willfully impeding relief supplies as provided for under the Geneva Conventions."); *See also* Elements of Crimes, International Criminal Court (2001), at art. 8(2)(b)(xxv), https://www.icc-cpi.int/nr/rdonlyres/336923d8-a6ad-40ec-ad7b-45bf9de73d56/0/elementsofcrimeseng.pdf.

3. The good effect must be produced directly by the action, not by the bad effect (i.e., it is not permitted to use a bad means to achieve a good end);

4. The good effect must be sufficiently desirable to compensate for allowing the bad effect (i.e. the good that is achieved must be proportional to the bad that is allowed).[26]

A campaign of starvation clearly fails the first condition because starvation is never morally good or morally indifferent. Even if the tactic of a blockade could be viewed as morally indifferent, if the effect of the blockade is to cause starvation, then the blockade fails the third condition because a bad effect (e.g., starvation) must never be used to achieve a good end (e.g., preventing weapons from entering enemy hands).

Part II: The use of starvation as a weapon of war is *malum in se*

The use of starvation as a method of war is *malum in se* because it violates the *jus in bello* principles of distinction, proportionality, necessity, and superfluous injury.

Starvation as a weapon of war violates the *jus in bello* principle of distinction.

Starvation is an inherently indiscriminate weapon. IHL requires that military attacks distinguish between civilians and combatants. When starvation is used lawfully, either through siege or blockade, it is impossible to distinguish between civilians and combatants. This is why the Additional Protocols require combatants to (1) allow humanitarian aid to be distributed to civilians during blockades and sieges and/or (2) allow civilians to leave besieged cities. Similarly, an otherwise lawful attack on enemy territory may cause starvation if the attack destroys OIS. Since water supplies and agricultural sites are used by both civilians and combatants, destruction of OIS intended to force capitulation of the enemy is also *malum in se* because such attacks are indiscriminate.

Some might argue that when used lawfully, starvation caused by sieges, blockades, or attacks on OIS that target combatants is not *malum in se* so long as civilian suffering is limited. To that end, the problem is not that sieges, blockades, or attacks on OIS cannot distinguish between civilians and combatants, but rather, combatants choose not to distinguish between

---

26. Stephen Coleman, *Military Ethics: An Introduction with Case Studies* (Oxford University Press 2012), 22.

civilians and combatants. These bad actors are thus violating the LOAC and should be punished in accordance with the Geneva Conventions or the Rome Statute.

The reality though, is that even "good"-intentioned combatants who undertake sieges, blockades, or attacks cannot absolutely guarantee that these tactics will not cause harm to civilians. In this way, methods of warfare that cause starvation fail to satisfy the fourth condition of DDE—namely, that the "good" effect of bringing about the capitulation of the enemy is not sufficiently desirable to compensate for allowing the bad effect of causing indiscriminate starvation of civilians. Moreover, in many, if not most cases, humanitarian aid does not reach civilians either because it is pilfered by belligerents or destroyed en route to civilians. And civilians are not always capable of leaving besieged cities. The elderly, disabled, and small children—to whom special duties of care are owed both legally and ethically—cannot be easily moved, and often there is nowhere else to go. Thus, even under the best of intentions, civilians suffer great harm when sieges, blockades, and attacks on OIS are used as a method of war. This is evidenced by the many instances of starvation during armed conflicts over the past 100 years, but especially in the recent conflicts in Sudan, Syria, and Yemen where hundreds of thousands of civilians have died due to starvation and related diseases because of war.[27]

Starvation as a weapon of war violates the *jus in bello* principle of proportionality.

Starvation often results in disproportionate casualties. The *jus in bello* principle of proportionality prohibits combatants from launching an attack or using means of warfare that *may* be expected to result in excessive civilian harm. Regardless of whether sieges, blockades, or attacks on OIS are lawful, they very often result in excessive civilian harm. The Nazi Hunger Plan led to the deaths of over four million people,[28] and the current civil war in Yemen has placed thirteen million people at risk of death or severe malnutrition and illness from starvation.[29] In the context of the Hunger Plan, where the Nazis planned to feed the German army by pillaging food from the Soviet

---

27. *See* Jennifer Trahan, *Existing Legal Limits to Security Council Veto Power in the Face of Atrocity Crimes*, 278–79 (Cambridge University Press 2020); *See also*, Laura Graham, "Pathways to Accountability for Starvation Crimes in Yemen," *Case Western J. of Intl. L.* 53 (2020).

28. De Waal, *supra* note 17, at 104.

29. BBC News, "Yemen could be 'worst famine in 100 years,'" (Oct. 15, 2018), https://www.bbc.com/news/av/world-middle-east-45857729.

Union, the starvation deaths of 4.7 million people is neither proportionate to a legitimate military objective, nor is it justified under DDE's second condition—that the agent must intend to bring about the good effect with the action and not a bad one. The Nazis did not intend a good effect. As I will show in the case study in part three, while one purpose of the Hunger Plan (feeding the German army) could be viewed as legitimate if other conditions were met, the primary purpose was to exterminate the Soviets. Extermination of a national or ethnic group is genocide, which is always *malum in se*. And concerning the thirteen million people at risk of starvation in Yemen due to blockades and attacks on OIS, even if a legitimate military objective is being pursued by these tactics, the sheer number of civilians at risk of death and disease (approximately 45% of the population),[30] is excessive and therefore not proportionate to a legitimate military objective.

A counterargument to the view that starvation as a method of war is disproportionate is that when used to hasten enemy capitulation, starvation may ultimately save innocent lives. To that end, many war historians believe that the use of starvation against the Germans during the first and second world wars escalated their capitulation, saving countless lives.[31] Some might argue that if such tactics bring about the capitulation of the enemy faster than a sustained military campaign, then we should consider the civilian casualties of sieges, blockades, and destruction of OIS as proportionate to what would have been a larger loss of life over a protracted conflict.

However, to better understand the loss of life due to starvation in the first and second world wars, one must broaden the timeframe. The civilian loss of life is not just the immediate days or months of a siege or blockade; rather, the loss of life must be calculated over the course of months and sometimes years of food insecurity and disease caused by the siege or blockade even after the war has ended. The "turnip winter" of 1916–17 in Germany, caused in part by US embargoes, led to the deaths of at least 750,000 Germans due to malnutrition, and the birth rate fell significantly.[32] Many of those deaths occurred during the six months *after* the armistice.[33] During World War II, at least twenty million people died from starvation,

---

30. The World Bank, "Total Population Yemen," https://data.worldbank.org/indicator/SP.POP.TOTL?locations=YE.
31. *See generally*, Lizzie Collingham, *The Taste of War: World War II and the Battle for Food* (2012).
32. *Id.* at 25.
33. De Waal, *supra* note 17, at 74.

malnutrition, and associated diseases.[34] Of those twenty million, one million died during the Siege of Leningrad.[35] In that context then, it is clear that the loss of civilian life is far greater than what would be permissible under the proportionality principle.

Starvation as a weapon of war violates the *jus in bello* principle of necessity.

Starvation is never necessary in war. The *jus in bello* principle of necessity permits measures that are *actually* necessary to accomplish a legitimate military purpose. Preventing weapons and other supplies from reaching enemy hands is a legitimate military purpose that may be achieved by a blockade. But, where blockades also prevent humanitarian aid from reaching civilians or allowing civilians access to food or water, those methods of war are morally impermissible because they cause unnecessary suffering and harm to civilians. And because a legitimate military purpose cannot be ethically achieved by means that are morally corrupt, starvation—whether it be a direct or indirect consequence of a legal method of warfare—will not satisfy the principle of necessity.

Opponents of absolute prohibitions on sieges, blockades, and other legal methods of warfare that employ the starvation tactic believe that such prohibitions would remove a vital weapon that militaries *may* need in certain rare cases. For example, where military defeat is inevitable *but for* the use of a siege of an enemy-combatant stronghold or a blockade to prevent flow of munitions to the enemy, then these means of warfare may be an *actual* necessity. Unlike rape or genocide, which are *mala in se* because they are *never* justified,[36] these opponents would argue that in certain rare cases, such as a "Supreme Emergency,"[37] starvation not only is the lesser evil, but it is also justified in order to prevent a worse tragedy or defeat. And when the legitimate needs of a military objective significantly outweigh civilian deaths by starvation, the use of starvation is justified under the necessity principle.

While there may be rare supreme emergencies that justify extreme measures to prevent human annihilation, in reality there will always be some alternative to sieges, blockades, and attacks on OIS. Under the second condition of DDE, the action is unjustified if the agent could attain the

---

34. Collingham, *supra* note 31, at 2.
35. *Id.* at 5.
36. *See* Morten Dige, *Explaining the Principle of Mala in Se, J. Mil. Ethics* 11(2012), 318–332, 319.
37. Michael Walzer, *Just and Unjust Wars*, 252 (1977).

good effect (military victory) without the bad effect (starvation). Moreover, in Orend's analysis, Walzer's concept of a supreme emergency corrupts the Just War tradition by dismissing the moral justifications of *jus in bello* requirements.[38] Applying this logic, starvation as a method of warfare could never be justified, even in a supreme emergency, because to permit such an evil act would bastardize the moral underpinnings of *jus in bello* principles. Thus, although starvation may be an efficient method of bringing the enemy to capitulation, it is not an actual military necessity even in the direst circumstances. Even if starvation as a method of warfare was *actually* necessary because of an existential threat, the suffering caused by such a method is evil in itself and must be absolutely prohibited. Therefore, the supreme emergency necessity argument is uncompelling because the starving of innocents is inherently evil and can never be justified under *jus in bello* requirements.[39]

Starvation as a weapon of war violates the *jus in bello* principle of superfluous injury.

Starvation causes superfluous injury or unnecessary harm to civilians and combatants alike. Much like landmines, cluster munitions, biological weapons, and other weapons that are illegal because of their pernicious effects, starvation as a tool of war is insidious. Death by starvation is an agonizing process. It takes the average human two full months to die from starvation.[40] According to food and war scholar Lizzie Collingham:

> Victims of starvation die of nutritional dystrophy, a process whereby, once the body has used up all its fat reserves, the muscles are broken down in order to obtain energy. The small intestine atrophies and it becomes increasingly difficult for the victim to absorb nutrients from what little food he or she is able to obtain. As a defence mechanism the body reduces the activity of the vital organs such as the heart and liver and the victim suffers not only from muscular debility but from a more general and overpowering fatigue.... The water content of the body reduces at a slower rate than the wasting of the muscles and tissues and the flaccidity of the body increases. Some victims of starvation

---

38. Brian Orend, *The Morality of War*, 147–148 (2006); *See also*, Martin Cook, "Michael Walzer's Concept of 'Supreme Emergency,'" *J. Mil. Ethics* 6 (2007):138–151, 143.
39. *See, e.g.,* Dige, *supra* note 36, at 319.
40. De Waal, *supra* note 17, at 21.

develop hunger oedema and swell up with excess water. The swelling begins in the abdomen and legs and spreads throughout the body. The skin becomes stretched, shiny and hypersensitive. Blood pressure drops and the victim is plagued by keratitis (redness and soreness of the cornea), sore gums, headaches, pains in the legs, neuralgic pains, tremors and ataxia (a loss of control over the limbs). The symptoms are accompanied by an intensive craving for carbohydrates and salt, and uncontrollable diarrhea. Just before death the victim veers wildly from depression to intense irritation and then a profound torpor. Eventually, the body has no alternative but to sustain itself by taking protein from the vital organs....Most importantly, the heart atrophies....Organ failure is the final cause of death.[41]

There is no military gain that can justify use of this pernicious weapon.

Some might argue that humankind has been using starvation as a weapon of war for millennia. If it were so terrible, it would no longer be permissible during war and perpetrators of starvation crimes would be prosecuted. Incidentally, no one has ever been punished for the crime of starvation. The lack of prohibitions and prosecutions may be evidence that the international community finds this tactic acceptable—or at least more acceptable than landmines, cluster munitions, and biological weapons. Additionally, an argument can be made that combatant deaths by starvation are no worse than death by bombing and other legal means of warfare. Indeed, because the purpose of sieges and blockades is not specifically to starve the enemy to death, but rather, to starve them into submission and surrender, the pernicious effects of starvation in the late stages of organ failure is an unlikely occurrence since the enemy will usually capitulate long before it gets to that stage.

This argument fails though because the lack of prosecutions of perpetrators of starvation crimes is a problem of political will and stalemate at the UN Security Council, and not a reflection of a lack of international perception of the horror of starvation. Just because the international community has not taken steps to end the blockades and attacks on OIS in Yemen, for example, does not mean that there have not been efforts to do so. The UN Security Council passed Resolution 2417 in an effort to condemn starvation as a result of the war in Yemen, and a 2019 amendment to Rome

---

41. Collingham, *supra* note 31, at 5–6.

Statute expands the war crime of starvation to apply to non-international armed conflicts.[42] The dearth of prosecutions for starvation crimes simply reflects the geopolitics of our current international order. While there may be no inevitable attempts to save Yemen, in the long run, the arc of justice is bending towards stricter and perhaps eventually absolute prohibitions on starvation as a method of war. Additionally, the idea that the enemy will capitulate before the pernicious effects of starvation take hold is not supported by historical evidence. Indeed, what tends to happen during sieges and blockades is that enemy combatants reserve vital food and water rations for themselves, furthering the plight of civilians in war zones. In fact, it is the civilians who suffer most during sieges and blockades because of limited quantities of food or water, lack of access to clean water, and because civilians are more likely to consist of the very young, the old, the infirm, and pregnant women, all of whom are less likely to be able to sustain a prolonged period of food shortage. Regardless of how many or how few die from starvation, the principle of superfluous harm prohibits unnecessary suffering, and death by starvation is an intolerably cruel way to die.

Part III: Starvation Case Studies: The Nazi Hunger Plan and Yemen's Civil War

Nazi Hunger Plan

It is well established that the Germans capitulated in World War I because they were starving and could no longer carry on military objectives without access to adequate food supplies.[43] As many as 750,000 Germans died as a result of malnutrition from the war.[44] In the lead up to World War II, the fact that so many Germans experienced starvation during the first world war was very much at the forefront of Hitler's concerns and plans for world domination.[45] Due to a combination of not wanting a repeat of Germany's defeat from World War I and the Nazi plan to expand the living space for Germans through the Lebensraum policy, the Nazis relied on the Reich

---

42. S.C. Res. 2417, ¶¶ 5–7 (May 24, 2018); International Criminal Court Assembly of State Parties, Report of the Working Group on Amendments, Eighteenth session, 2–7 December 2019, 7–9, ICC-ASP/18/32 (Dec. 3, 2019), https://asp.icc-cpi.int/iccdocs/asp_docs/ASP18/ICC-ASP-18-32-ENG.pdf.
43. *Id. See also,* Alex De Waal, *supra* note 17, at 74; Gesine Gerhard, "Food and Genocide: Nazi Agrarian Politics in the Occupied Territories of the Soviet Union," *Contemporary European History* 18, 45–65.
44. De Waal, *supra* note 17.
45. *Id.* at 75.

Ministry of Food and Agriculture to develop policies to address food shortages and rationing to help the Nazis achieve victory in the war.[46] While much of the work of the Ministry in the early part of the war was to increase food production in Germany and Nazi-occupied territories as well as ration food for German civilians and soldiers, the Ministry was also responsible for setting the caloric requirements for Holocaust victims in concentration camps as well as POWs.[47] Nazi victims were allowed a mere 184 to 845 calories a day—a starvation diet.[48]

By 1941, it was clear that in order for the Nazis to defeat the Red Army and pursue global domination, the Wehrmacht (German Army) would need a steady supply of food, which was not available in Germany.[49] The Nazis calculated that each of the 9.5 million men in the army would need to eat 3,000 calories a day to carry out military activities.[50] By 1943, the Wehrmacht was consuming 40% of the total grain and 62% of the total meat available to the Reich, leading to food shortages for civilians in Germany.[51] The most valuable weapon of war, therefore, was food.

Fearing a repeat of Germany's defeat in World War I, the Nazis developed a plan that would help them defeat the Red Army and provide ample food to Germans for the duration of the war.[52] In March–May 1941, a series of high-level meetings took place between Herbert Backe, the author of the Hunger Plan; Hermann Göring, Plenipotentiary of the Four-Year Plan and Supreme Commander of the Luftwaffe (Air Force); Adolf Hitler; and other high-ranking Nazi leaders regarding the Nazi Party's Four-Year Plan for victory.[53] The result of those meetings was a plan to starve thirty million "useless eaters" in the Soviet Union.[54] The Hunger Plan identified surplus zones of food production and deficit zones in the Soviet Union.[55] The surplus zones—predominantly Ukraine, known as the granary of the Soviet Union, as well as southern Russia and the Caucasus region, were to be captured by the Wehrmacht and used to send 8.7 million tons of surplus

---

46. *Id.* at 101.

47. Collingham, *supra* note 31, at 4–5.

48. *Id.*

49. *Id.* at 179–180.

50. *Id.* at 180.

51. *Id.*

52. De Waal, *supra* note 17, at 102; Gerhard, *supra* note 43, at 46–47.

53. Alex J. Kay, *Exploitation, Resettlement, Mass Murder: Political and Economic Planning for German Occupation Policy in the Soviet Union, 1940–1941,* 47–67 (2011 e-book).

54. De Waal, *supra* note 17, at 102; Gerhard, *supra* note 43, at 46.

55. Gerhard, *supra* note 43, at 56–57.

food to Germany, while the deficit zones—large urban centers like Moscow in northern and central Russia that required food be brought in, were to be cut off from all food supplies in order to exterminate the population.[56] The result of the policy, had it fully succeeded, would have led to the starvation of thirty million Slavic and Jewish people in the Soviet Union.[57]

In May 1941, the Nazis held a conference in Wannsee, a small lake town just outside Berlin. Following the Wannsee Conference, a twenty-page document from the Economic Policy Guidelines for Economic Organization East outlining the Hunger Plan was circulated to top Nazi officials.[58] It noted:

> The population of these territories, in particular the population of the cities will have to face the most terrible famine.... Many tens of millions of people in this territory will become superfluous and will die or must emigrate to Siberia. Attempts to reduce the population there from death through starvation by obtaining surpluses from the black earth zone can only be at the expense of the provisioning of Europe. They prevent the possibility of Germany holding out till the end of the war, they prevent Germany and Europe from resisting the blockade.[59]

The Nazis formalized their starvation plan and then instigated the worst starvation crime in history.[60]

The Nazis pursued the Hunger Plan under the guise of Operation Barbarossa—the Axis invasion of the Soviet Union.[61] But the Nazis miscalculated the scale of the offensive, and were ultimately unable to achieve victory against the Red Army due to attrition—i.e., the Red Army had worn down the Wehrmacht through continuous losses of soldiers.[62] The Nazis severely underestimated the difficulty of defeating the Red Army, which outnumbered the Wehrmacht by 2:1.[63] Despite miscalculating the Red Army's strength, the

56. *Id. See also*, Kay, *supra* note 53, at 127.
57. De Waal, *supra* note 17, at 102–3.
58. Gerhard, *supra* note 43, at 58.
59. Kay, *supra* note 53, at 135.
60. De Waal, *supra* note 17, at 15.
61. *Id.* at 102.
62. Holocaust Encyclopedia, "Invasion of the Soviet Union, June 1941, US Holocaust Memorial Museum," https://encyclopedia.ushmm.org/content/en/article/invasion-of-the-soviet-union-june-1941.
63. Reina Pennington, "Was the Russian Military a Steamroller? From World War II to Today," *War on the Rocks* (Jul. 6, 2016), https://warontherocks.com/2016/07/was-the-russian-military-a-steamroller-from-world-war-ii-to-today/.

Nazis did achieve a small fraction of their intended purpose in the Hunger Plan—Operation Barbarossa led to the deaths of one million Soviets due to starvation during the 900-day Siege of Leningrad.[64] A further 1–2 million Soviet POWs were starved to death in Nazi labor camps.[65]

One of the primary reasons the Hunger Plan failed in its principal objective is because the Nazis underestimated the difficulty and time needed to starve thirty million people. It takes two months of no food for the average human being to starve to death.[66] For example, the IRA Hunger Striker Bobby Sands died without food after sixty-six days.[67] But the Nazis were never able to completely cut off the food supply in the Soviet Union, in part, due to the availability of food on the black market.[68] And so it took much longer to starve the population, all the while trying to defeat the Red Army through combat. It was too much to achieve, and eventually the Nazis retreated.[69] The Nazi Hunger Plan, which planned to kill thirty million people, ultimately killed around 4.7 million.[70] Had it succeeded, it would have been the worst atrocity ever committed.

Despite the fact that 4.7 million people were starved to death under the Hunger Plan, neither Herbert Backe, Hermann Göring, nor Walter Darré (Reich Minister of Food and Agriculture during the Hunger Plan) were ever charged with violating the laws of war with respect to starvation of civilians as a method of warfare. The reasons for this relate to the custom of the time, which did not prohibit starvation as a method of warfare. However, as I have argued above, the use of starvation as a weapon of the Nazi Hunger Plan is *malum in se* both because it can never be morally or ethically justified by the principles of IHL, and because it fails all four conditions of the DDE. It fails the first condition because weaponized starvation is neither morally good nor morally indifferent. It fails the second condition because the Nazis' intention was never to bring about a good effect, but rather, to exterminate 30 million Soviets while feeding the German army.

---

64. Collingham, *supra* note 31, at 5.
65. *Id.* at 193; Gerhard, *supra* note 43, at 60–61.
66. Collingham, *supra* note 31, at 5–6; De Waal, *supra* note 17, at 21.
67. *Id.*
68. Kay, *supra* note 53, at 134–35.
69. Encyclopedia Britannica Online, "Stalingrad and the German retreat, summer 1942–February 1943," https://www.britannica.com/event/World-War-II/Stalingrad-and-the-German-retreat-summer-1942-February-1943.
70. De Waal, *supra* note 17, at 104 (noting that it is impossible to know exactly how high the death toll of the Hunger Plan was, but settling on the figure 4.7 million on the basis of leading historians' calculations).

The third condition fails because starvation of over 4 million people is a bad effect lacking justification. And the fourth condition fails because the arguable "good" effect—diverting food from the Soviet Union to feed the German army—cannot compensate for the bad effect of starving 4.7 million people. Thus, the Hunger Plan is unjustified under the principles of IHL and it fails the DDE.

Yemen's Civil War

The war in Yemen has created the world's worst humanitarian crisis.[71] Due to the ongoing civil war that began in 2015 between Houthi rebels and the Yemeni government, widespread hunger and disease have left tens of thousands of civilians dead. More than twenty million people are suffering from food insecurity and preventable diseases such as cholera and severe malnutrition.[72] Since 2017, an estimated thirteen million Yemenis have been declared at risk of starvation[73] and at least 85,000 children have died from starvation and starvation-related diseases.[74] Yemen has been teetering on the brink of famine since before the war broke out in 2015.

As the poorest nation in the Middle East, approximately 44% of Yemenis were undernourished in 2012, with as many as five million people relying on emergency food aid.[75] Water scarcity was such a significant problem for this

71. Remarks by the Secretary-General to the Pledging Conference on Yemen, The United Nations Office at Geneva (Apr. 1, 2018), https://www.unog.ch/unog/website/news_media. nsf/(httpNewsByYear_en)/27F6CCAD7178F3E9C1258264003311FA?OpenDocument; *See also* Stephen O'Brien, Statement to the Security Council on Missions to Yemen, South Sudan, Somalia, and Kenya and an Update on the Oslo Conference on Nigeria and the Lake Chad Region, United Nations Security Council (Mar. 10, 2017) https://docs.unocha. org/sites/dms/Documents/ERC_USG_Stephen_OBrien_Statement_to_the_SecCo_on_ Missions_to_Yemen_South_Sudan_Somalia_and_Kenya_and_update_on_Oslo.pdf (Head of United Nations Office Stephen O'Brien telling the Security Council "We stand at a critical point in history. Already at the beginning of the year we are facing the largest humanitarian crisis since the creation of the United Nations.") [hereinafter, O'Brien Statement 2017].
72. Humanitarian Aid, "Humanitarian crisis in Yemen remains the worst in the world, warns UN," *UN News* (Feb. 14, 2019), https://news.un.org/en/story/2019/02/1032811; Doctors Without Borders/Médecins Sans Frontières
(MSF) has treated 143,467 cholera and 23,319 malnutrition cases between March 2015 and September 2019. *See* Médecins Sans Frontières, "Yemen: Crisis Update November 2019," https://www.doctorswithoutborders.org/what-we-do/news-stories/story/yemen-crisis-update-november-2019.
73. BBC News, "Yemen could be 'worst famine in 100 years,'" (Oct. 15, 2018), https://www.bbc.com/news/av/world-middle-east-45857729.
74. Bethan McKernan, "Yemen: up to 85,000 young children dead from starvation," *The Guardian* (Nov. 21, 2018), https://www.theguardian.com/world/2018/nov/21/yemen-young-children-dead-starvation-disease-save-the-children.
75. Joseph Hincks, "What you need to know about the crisis in Yemen," *Time* (Nov. 3, 2016), https://time.com/4552712/yemen-war-humanitarian-crisis-famine/.

arid country that in 2012 experts predicted that the country's water would run out by 2017.[76] In early 2017, the UN declared Yemen in danger of imminent famine.[77] A famine is "a crisis of mass hunger that causes elevated mortality over a specific period of time"[78] and have multiple causes that include "both structural factors that determine vulnerability and the proximate triggers of the crisis."[79] Famines can be distinguished by magnitude (the number of casualties) and severity (the level of food insecurity).[80] The severity of food insecurity consists of five phases: (1) minimal; (2) stressed; (3) crisis; (4) emergency; and (5) famine.[81] Multiple regions in Yemen are presently described as being in phase 3 crisis or phase 4 emergency.[82] The worst areas of food insecurity are where the conflict is being fought—Hudaydah, Sana'a, Ta'izz, Aden, and the Red Sea Coast villages.

Civilian deaths in Yemen caused by starvation and starvation-related diseases such as cholera are man-made.[83] Two categories of events are primarily responsible for starvation deaths and injury: (1) military attacks on agricultural and food production that destroy, deny, or render useless OIS, and (2) blockades of airports and seaports causing obstruction of humanitarian aid.[84] The groups responsible for these atrocities include all of the major parties to the conflict: Iranian-supported Houthi rebels, Yemeni government and military, as well as the Saudi Arabia-led Coalition (SLC). Documentation of attacks on civilian food supplies shows that perpetrators targeted civilians as part of

---

76. Frederika Whitehead, Water scarcity in Yemen: the country's forgotten conflict, *The Guardian* (Apr. 2, 2015, 5:18 a.m.), https://www.theguardian.com/global-development-professionals-network/2015/apr/02/water-scarcity-yemen-conflict; IRIN in Sana'a, "Time running out for solution to Yemen's water crisis," *The Guardian* (Aug. 27, 2912, 7:30 a.m.), https://www.theguardian.com/global-development/2012/aug/27/solution-yemen-water-crisis.

77. O'Brien Statement 2017, *supra* note 71.

78. Alex De Waal, "The end of famine? Prospects for the elimination of mass starvation by political action," *Political Geography* 62 (2018): 184, 185

79. *Id.* at 185.

80. Paul Howe and Stephen Deveraux, "Famine Intensity and Magnitude Scales: A proposal for an instrumental definition of famine," *Disasters* 28 (2004): 353–372; Famine Early Warning Systems Network, Integrated Phase Classification, https://fews.net/IPC.

81. Famine Early Warning Systems Network, "Integrated Phase Classification," https://fews.net/IPC.

82. Famine Early Warning Systems Network, "Yemen Food Security Outlook," October 2019 to May 2020, https://fews.net/east-africa/yemen/food-security-outlook/october-2019.

83. *See generally* De Waal, *supra* note 17.

84. Martha Mundy, "The Strategies of the Coalition in the Yemen War: Aerial Bombardment and Food War," *World Peace Foundation* 11 (2018), https://sites.tufts.edu/wpf/files/2018/10/Strategies-of-Coalition-in-Yemen-War-Final-20181005-1.pdf [hereinafter Mundy].

a method of warfare, an unambiguous violation of *jus in bello* and Just War tradition.[85] Some reports point to Saudi Arabia's Crown Prince Mohammad bin Salman having authorized the use of starvation as a method of warfare to defeat the Houthis.[86]

One of the main contributors to starvation and related diseases in Yemen has been the deliberate and disproportionate destruction of OIS, which includes attacks on critical infrastructure such as electricity sources, water supplies, irrigation dams, agricultural extension facilities, and health facilities. The Human Rights Council reported that SLC airstrikes have caused significant damage to civilian objects, leading to numerous civilian deaths.[87] Destruction of OIS in Ta'izz, Tihama, and the Red Sea Coast are some of the most egregious incidents of the war in Yemen causing starvation of civilians.

Because it was one of the primary battlegrounds in the conflict between Houthi rebels and the SLC, the Ta'izz governorate suffered some of the worst death tolls of the war. Beginning in 2014, civilian objects were repeatedly targeted, leading to the deaths and displacement of many civilians.[88] A variety of factors have worsened food insecurity in Ta'izz, leading to starvation of civilians. As a result of ongoing fighting, access to food in markets has been reduced significantly, and the price of food items has increased drastically, making food unaffordable for many.[89] Additionally, SLC airstrikes targeting farms, markets, agricultural offices, and transportation centers have further increased food shortages.[90] In December 2017, SLC airstrikes targeted a market in al-Ta'iziyah district, completely destroying the market and leaving fifty-four civilians dead and a further thirty-two injured.[91] Seventy five percent of the civilian population in

---

85. *Id.* at 24.
86. A senior Saudi Arabia-led Coalition Arabia-led Coalition diplomat stated off-record, "Once we control them, we will feed them." *Id.* at 7; *See also* "Bin Salman threatens to target women and children in Yemen despite international criticism," *Middle East Monitor* (Aug. 27, 2018, 10:39 a.m.), https://www.middleeastmonitor.com/20180827-bin-salman-threatens-to-target-women-and-children-in-yemen-despite-international-criticism/.
87. UN Office of the High Commissioner on Human Rights, Yemen: United Nations Experts point to possible war crimes by parties to the conflict (Aug. 28, 2018), https://www.ohchr.org/EN/NewsEvents/Pages/DisplayNews.aspx?NewsID=23479.
88. World Peace Foundation, Accountability for Mass Starvation: Starvation in Yemen Policy Brief, World Peace Foundation, 6–7 (2019), https://sites.tufts.edu/wpf/files/2019/06/Accountability-for-Starvation-Crimes-Yemen.pdf [hereinafter WPF Policy Brief].
89. *Id.* at 6–7.
90. *Id.*
91. *Id.*

Ta'izz in August 2018 were ranked as food insecure and at least 85% were dependent on humanitarian aid.[92]

In addition to the attacks in Ta'izz, other areas of the country, including fishing villages, have been targeted. Many airstrikes on agricultural targets were conducted from March 2015 to August 2016.[93] Attacks on agricultural land are particularly egregious because only 5% of Yemen's land is arable, and prior to the war, only 3% of Yemen's total land surface was used for agriculture.[94] In Tihama, the attacks on OIS were not on fields or flocks, but on irrigation systems powered by oil-driven pumping. Beginning in 2011, and as a consequence of the war, oil shortages and price increases have made it nearly impossible for farmers to irrigate their land.[95]

Since the late 1970s, the World Bank has invested in professionally engineered water diversion structures, overseen by the Tihama Development Authority (TDA), used to strengthen water disbursement to farm lands in the region.[96] Twice in August 2015 and again in September, the SLC delivered a total of fifteen airstrikes on the TDA's central compound just outside Hudaydah, and a further three airstrikes attacked irrigation structures in Wadi Siham in October 2015.[97] The Yemen Data Project reports two additional attacks on TDA infrastructure in 2016 and another three in early 2017.[98] As a consequence of these attacks, agricultural yields decreased by 24% among farmers in Wadi Zabid and 46% in Wadi Siham, due primarily to irrigation water shortages.[99] The Tihama region, once considered the breadbasket of Yemen, has decreased land cultivation by 51%, crop yields declined by 20–61% per hectare, and there has been a complete annihilation of fruits, vegetables, and livestock population, leading to 43% of the population being food insecure.[100]

---

92. *Id.*

93. Mundy, *supra* note 84, at 11.

94. Food and Agriculture Organization of the United Nations, "Selected Indicators," http://www.fao.org/faostat/en/?#country/249.

95. Mundy, *supra* note 84, at 13.

96. *Id.* at 14.

97. *Id.*

98. *Id.*

99. The Water and Environment Center of San'a' University, *Food Production, Irrigation, Marketing, and Agricultural Coping Mechanisms, Tihama* (Wadi Zabid and Wadi Siham), Briefing Note 2-Food Security (FBLN, NICHE-Yem027), Flood-Based Livelihoods Network Foundation, http://spate-irrigation-org/wp-content/uploads/2018/02/Briefing-Note-2-%E2%80%93-Food-Security-pdf.

100. Flood-based Livelihoods Network Foundation, "Yemen's Burnt Granary," http://spate-irrigation.org/yemens-burnt-granary/#more-6422.

Artisanal fishing has long been a primary source of food production in Yemen. The General Authority of Fishing in the Red Sea documented damages to fishing from the beginning of the war through December 2017, reporting 146 fishermen killed and 220 fishing boats destroyed by SLC airstrikes in 2018.[101] Prior to the war in 2015, Yemen's fisheries sector ranked second in terms of exports and constituted 2% of Yemen's GDP.[102]

Another major cause of starvation in Yemen is the unlawful obstruction and manipulation of humanitarian relief because of blockades. Evidence of impeding humanitarian supplies and operations shows that blockades have halted delivery of humanitarian assistance and have caused unreasonable delays in transportation of humanitarian aid to areas affected by the famine.

Hudaydah was Yemen's poorest governorate prior to the outbreak of war in 2015.[103] Sixty percent of Yemen's malnourished population resided in Hudaydah.[104] There are three major ports in the governorate, two of which (Al-Hudaydah and Al-Saleef) receive the majority of Yemen's food imports; the total number of commercial imports has declined significantly since 2014.[105] There are two other ports in Yemen at Aden and Al-Mukalla, but they lack the infrastructure necessary to receive bulk food shipments.[106] In April 2015, the SLC undertook a blockade of the Red Sea ports in order to inspect commercial ships that could be carrying prohibited weapons to the Houthis.[107] The consequence of the blockade, which lasted sixteen months, was to effectively limit the flow of food, fuel, and medicine to civilians.[108] On 6 November 2017, the SLC retaliated against a Houthi missile attack on Riyadh by imposing a sixteen-day total air, sea, and land blockade of Yemen, which blocked all food and fuel coming into the country,[109] leading to increased food insecurity and deaths by starvation and malnutrition.

The war in Yemen presents a very different case study from the Nazi Hunger Plan. While the Nazis used starvation as a weapon of extermina-

---

101. Taqrir 'an al-qita ' al-samaki fi-'l-bahr al-ahmar ba'd alf yaum min al-'udwan [Report on the fishing sector in the Red Sea after a thousand days of the aggression] al-Hai'ah al-'Amman li'-Masa'id al-Samakiya fi'l-Bahr al-Ahmar, 13–43 (Jan. 2018).
102. Ammar Al-Fareh, "The Impact of the War in Yemen on Artisanal Fishing of the Red Sea," *LSE Middle East Centre Report* 7 (2018), http://eprints.lse.ac.uk/91022/1/Al-Fareh_The-impact-of-war_Author.pdf.
103. WPF Policy Brief, *supra* note 88, at 7.
104. *Id.*
105. *Id.*
106. *Id.* at 7–8.
107. *Id.*
108. *Id.* at 8.
109. *Id.*

tion, the SLC are using blockades and attacks on Houthi-strongholds. Even if it could be proven that the SLC's tactics did not intentionally starve civilians or specifically target OIS for destruction, which would be very difficult to prove based on the evidence presented above, these tactics are nevertheless *malum in se* because the result is reckless indifference to the starvation of civilians in violation of the four principles of IHL set forth above. Additionally, although SLC blockades and airstrikes in Yemen may intend a good effect (e.g., to defeat the Houthi rebels and restore peace and security in the region), the bad effect (starvation) fails justification under DDE's third and fourth conditions because it is impermissible to use a bad means to achieve a good end, and the effect of bringing an end to the war, which has not worked anyway, is not proportional to the starvation deaths of civilians. For these reasons, I advocate for stricter prohibitions on legal methods of warfare that lead either directly or indirectly to starvation.

Part IV: Conclusion

This paper has argued that the use of starvation as a method of warfare should be absolutely prohibited under international law because it is *malum in se*. While some might argue that both IHL and ICL prohibit starvation already, I submit that the current legal instruments prohibiting starvation are inadequate, both because they are not enforced and because current instruments permit starvation when it is an indirect consequence of legal methods of warfare, such as sieges and blockades. These problems underscore the need for greater restrictions in the existing legal framework to ensure that starvation is never a permissible outcome of a military objective, whether directly or indirectly.

The problem of enforcement owes largely to the fact that the most recent examples where starvation crimes have been committed—Yemen and Syria—do not come under the jurisdiction of the ICC. Without a referral from the UN Security Council to the ICC, it is highly unlikely that perpetrators of starvation crimes will be held accountable[110] because the legal systems of these failed states are either unable or unwilling to prosecute perpetrators. Thus, the best that can be done is to preserve evidence of starvation crimes for future prosecutions and for the international community to put pressure on members of the Security Council, but in particular the P3 (US, China, and Russia), to pass a Chapter VII Resolution

---

110. Graham, *supra* note 27.

to investigate starvation crimes in Yemen and Syria, and to recommend prosecutions of those individuals.

Another way to bring an end to the use of starvation as a weapon of war is for states to make declarations condemning it and calling for the codification or progressive development of international law to place stricter prohibitions on starvation. Some strategies for pursuing this aim include characterizing the crime of starvation as a non-derogable *jus cogens* peremptory norm under existing treaties and conventions,[111] and lobbying for the Security Council to adopt a Chapter VII Resolution calling for an end to starvation as a weapon of war and describing it as *malum in se*. These steps would send a clear signal that starvation will no longer be tolerated under international law.

Finally, military ethicists can influence a change in the law by persuading state officials and military leaders that legal methods of warfare that cause starvation, whether directly or indirectly, are not necessary to achieve military objectives. Other means can achieve similar goals without the insidious consequences of civilian suffering caused by starvation. Thus, a shift in attitude among military leaders and state officials can create a new custom that starvation is *malum in se*, making it easier to place more meaningful legal restrictions on the use of starvation during war and ending impunity for perpetrators of starvation crimes.

---

111. The International Law Commission's work on *jus cogens* peremptory norms of general international law does not list the prohibition on starvation in its recent report, but the prohibition on crimes against humanity and genocide are certainly closely related to starvation. *See* Int'l Law Com., Peremptory norms of general international law (*jus cogens*), Text of the draft conclusions and draft annex provisionally adopted by the Drafting Committee on first reading, (May 29, 2019), A/CN.4/L.936.

Malum in se
Los crímenes de hambre en el derecho internacional

Laura K. Graham

Desde tiempos inmemoriales, el hambre ha sido utilizada como un método de guerra. Incluso, a pesar de la evolución en el derecho de los conflictos armados (DCA) en los últimos 150 años que se ha abocado a la prohibición de la utilización del hambre en los civiles durante la guerra, su uso persiste como método de guerra. Esto se debe a que los beligerantes cuentan con dos medios legales para utilizar el hambre: (1) el sitio de guerra y (2) los bloqueos destinados a cortar los suministros del enemigo. En el presente ensayo, sostengo que incluso cuando los beligerantes empleen el hambre para efectos de la guerra bajo la óptica del derecho internacional humanitario (DIH), tales tácticas nunca se justifican moralmente y deben prohibirse en su totalidad, puesto que la provocación del hambre es un acto *malum in se*, es decir, es un acto inmoral por naturaleza, independientemente de si el DIH lo prohíbe estrictamente. Esto es así porque cuando se utiliza como arma de guerra, el hambre viola los principios del *jus in bello*.

En la parte I, estudio el desarrollo histórico tanto del DIH como del derecho internacional penal (DIP) en relación con las prohibiciones, o más bien los permisos, sobre la utilización del hambre durante los conflictos armados comenzando con el Código Lieber de 1863 y terminando con la enmienda de 2019 al Estatuto de Roma, la cual prohíbe el hacer padecer hambre en conflictos armados sin carácter internacional y la define como un crimen de guerra. En la parte II, expongo mis argumentos de que el hambre es un acto *malum in se,* puesto que viola los principios del *jus in bello* sobre la distinción, la proporcionalidad, la necesidad y el daño superfluo. En la parte III, presento dos casos de estudio, uno histórico y otro contemporáneo, en los que se utiliza el hambre como arma de guerra. Primero, presento el Plan del Hambre de los nazis para destacar la postura inmoral de utilizar el hambre en contra del enemigo. Después, muestro el caso contemporáneo de la guerra civil en Yemen, donde trece millones de personas están en riesgo de morir de hambre o fallecer por enfermedades relacionadas con el hambre debido a los ataques de la Coalición liderada por Arabia Saudita contra la agricultura, el agua y los bienes indispensables para la supervivencia (BIS). Estos casos de estudio demuestran que incluso bajo el cobijo legal, el uso del hambre como arma de guerra es *malum in se* y debe prohibirse totalmente y castigarse conforme al derecho internacional. Por último, mi conclusión aboga a favor de prohibiciones más estrictas con respecto al hambre en virtud del derecho internacional, aunadas a algunas estrategias para que se cumpla este objetivo.

Parte I. Acontecimientos históricos relativos a la prohibición del hambre como método de guerra

Las leyes de la guerra, *jus in bello* o derecho internacional humanitario, rigen la conducta de las partes de un conflicto armado así como las tácticas militares que son permisibles en una guerra justa.[1] Entre las reglas humanitarias básicas de la guerra durante los siglos XIX y XX estaban los principios de necesidad militar y de proporcionalidad, la idea de que las partes de un conflicto armado pueden iniciar un ataque cuando sea realmente necesario para lograr un propósito militar legítimo, pero debe equilibrarse con el principio de proporcionalidad para reducir al máximo el daño a los civiles.[2] El tratado de Oppenheim, de *Derecho Internacional*, describe el primer y el segundo principio de las leyes de la guerra -necesidad y humanidad- como una contradicción que debe conciliarse.[3] Así pues, el derecho internacional humanitario, en su forma de reglamentos y convenios, fue elaborado para conciliar las necesidades de la guerra con el principio de humanidad.

---

1. En general, se considera que el derecho internacional humanitario se desarrolló después de que Henry Durant presenciara la Batalla de Solferino en 1859 y estableciera el movimiento de la Cruz Roja. El Código Lieber es considerado como el primer ejemplo de codificación de las leyes de la guerra. Sin embargo, las leyes de la guerra y el derecho internacional humanitario, aunque a menudo se utilicen indistintamente, son en realidad, distintas: el Derecho de Ginebra, derivado de los primeros Convenios de Ginebra, representa las costumbres de los principios humanitarios, mientras que el Derecho de La Haya, derivado de las Conferencias de Paz de La Haya de 1899 y 1907, representa las normas convencionales de la conducta de guerra. La mayoría de los juristas ya no consideran el Derecho de La Haya y el de Ginebra como distintos. Véase: Amanda Alexander, "A Short History of International Humanitarian Law," [Breve historia del derecho internacional humanitario] *European J. of Int'l L.* 26 (2015): 109, 112–116.

2. *Véase, por ejemplo,* Judith Gardam, *Necessity, Proporcionality and the Use of Force by States* [Necesidad, proporcionalidad y uso de la fuerza de los estados] (Cambridge University Press 2004 e-book) 28–30 (donde se explica que la necesidad y la proporcionalidad habían formado parte de la teoría de la guerra justa desde la Edad Media); Orden General No. 100 (24 de abril de 1863) Código Lieber, Instrucciones para el Gobierno de los Ejércitos de los Estados Unidos en el Campo de Batalla, Arts. 14–16, https://avalon.law.yale.edu/19th_century/lieber.asp#sec1 [en lo sucesivo, Código Lieber].

3. *Véase, por ejemplo,* L. Oppenheim, *International Law: A Treatise* [El derecho internacional: un tratado], editado por R. F. Roxburgh, 3ra ed. (1921), 84–85.

Las prohibiciones sobre el uso *innecesario* del hambre como método de guerra se remontan al Código Lieber de 1863, el cual reconoce que el hambre del enemigo es permisible para dar celeridad a la capitulación, pero que las muertes de civiles deben cumplir con los principios de necesidad y proporcionalidad del DIH, es decir, las muertes de civiles deben ser necesarias y proporcionales con un objetivo militar legítimo, como el poner fin a la guerra.[4] El Código Lieber, elaborado para el Ejército de la Unión de Estados Unidos durante la Guerra Civil, establece que:

> La guerra no sólo se ejecuta con armas. Es lícito matar de hambre al beligerante hostil, así esté armado o desarmado, si eso conduce a someter más rápidamente al enemigo. Cuando un comandante de un lugar sitiado expulsa a los no combatientes, con el fin de disminuir el número de consumidores de su inventario de provisiones, *es lícito, aunque se trate de una medida extrema para hacerlos retroceder a fin de expeditar su rendición.*[5]

Inherente a este código es la necesidad militar de utilizar el hambre para el acelerar la capitulación. El recurso del sitio o bloqueo debe llevarse a cabo para satisfacer una necesidad militar legítima, en otras palabras, no sería legítimo utilizar el hambre para castigar al enemigo, exterminar a la población o saquear el territorio del enemigo en busca de alimentos y suministros para mantener una campaña militar prolongada. Aunque el Código Lieber no menciona la proporcionalidad de manera expresa, podría interpretarse que el Artículo 18 la establece en tanto que el propósito de permitir la guerra de sitios sea acelerar la rendición, limitando así el número total de víctimas de la guerra. Lo que el Código Lieber no contempla es el principio de humanidad: que el sufrimiento, de los civiles en particular, es inadmisible e injusto. Por ello, sería exagerado proclamar que el Código Lieber fuera la primera codificación sobre la prohibición del uso del hambre en civiles, sin embargo, dadas las condiciones de necesidad militar y proporcionalidad implícitas en los Artículos 17 y 18, podría considerarse como un primer paso para ese propósito.

---

4. Código Lieber, nota *supra 3*, en Arts. 17-18
5. Código Lieber, nota *supra 3*, en Arts. 17-18 (énfasis añadido). Los permisos del Código Lieber para conducir a los combatientes de regreso a una zona sitiada a fin de acelerar la derrota del enemigo contrastan profundamente con la convención moderna de que, cuando sea posible, debe permitirse que las personas civiles y los no combatientes abandonen una zona sitiada o por lo menos permitir, que la ayuda humanitaria llegue a los civiles a pesar del sitio. *Véase, por ejemplo,* el Protocolo Adicional a los Convenios de Ginebra del 12 de agosto de 1949 relativo a la Protección de Víctimas de los Conflictos Armados Internacionales (Protocolo I), de 8 de junio de 1977, Arts. 54, 70

Aunque no existían prohibiciones expresas sobre el uso del hambre en los civiles en el siglo XIX, la Convención de La Haya de 1899 podría interpretarse a favor de la prevención del hambre en los civiles en virtud de la Cláusula de Martens, la cual prohíbe aquellos métodos de guerra que conmocionen la conciencia pública.[6] La Cláusula de Martens, expresada en el preámbulo de la Convención II de La Haya de 1899, dispone:

> Hasta que se dicte un código más completo de las leyes de la guerra, las Altas Partes Contratantes juzgan como justo el declarar que, en los casos no comprendidos en los reglamentos que estas hayan adoptado, *las poblaciones y los beligerantes permanecerán bajo el amparo y el régimen de los principios del derecho internacional*, cuales fueren los usos establecidos entre las naciones civilizadas, *de las leyes de la humanidad y de las exigencias de la conciencia pública.*[7]

El principio de humanidad desempeña una función de seguridad para evitar que los beligerantes se enfrasquen en una guerra antihumanitaria. Prohíbe todo método de guerra que sea innecesario para obtener una ventaja militar específica,[8] y está estrechamente vinculado con el principio que prohíbe aquellas armas que causen daños superfluos.[9] Jean Pictet interpretó el principio de humanidad en el sentido de que "los [no] combatientes serán perdonados en la medida de lo posible".[10] Una interpretación amplia es que, aun cuando un tratado o convención no prohíba de manera expresa, un acto o una conducta de los beligerantes, no implica que ese acto o esa conducta se permita de *ipso facto.* Más bien, ese acto o esa conducta están

---

6. El principio de humanidad, al que en ocasiones se hace referencia como la Cláusula de Martens, protege a los civiles de faltas al DIH que, de manera expresa, no se contemplan en los tratados. Fue introducido por Fiódor Fiódorovich Martens durante el preámbulo de la Convención de La Haya de 1899. *Véase:* CICR, "Principios fundamentales del DIH", https://casebook.icrc.org/glossary/fundamental-prin Principles-ihl.

7. Convenio (II) relativo a las leyes y costumbres de la guerra terrestre y sus anexos: Reglamento relativo a las leyes y costumbres de la guerra terrestre, La Haya, 29 de julio de 1899, Preámbulo (énfasis añadido).

8. E. Kwakwa, *The International Law of Armed Conflict: Personal and Material Fields of Application* [El derecho internacional de los conflictos armados; campos de aplicación personales y materiales] (Kluwer Academic, Dordrecht, 1992), 36.

9. Convenio (II) relativo a las leyes y costumbres de la guerra terrestre y su anexo: Reglamento relativo a las leyes y costumbres de la guerra terrestre, La Haya, 29 de julio de 1899, Preámbulo.

10. Jean Pictet, *Development and Principles of International Humanitarian Law* [Desarrollo y principios del derecho internacional humanitario], Martinus Nijhoff y Henry Dunant Institute (Dordrecht/Ginebra, 1985), 62.

sujetos a los principios del derecho internacional consuetudinario.[11] En el contexto del hambre provocada puede argumentarse que aunque ningún tratado o convención prohibió expresamente su uso en los civiles durante la Segunda Guerra Mundial, el principio de humanidad de Martens sugiere que si la utilización del hambre como método de guerra no cumplía un objetivo militar legítimo o no era proporcionado, entonces no era lícito, según las costumbres de la época.

Además, la Convención de La Haya de 1907 no menciona de manera expresa el hambre como método de guerra, pero dispone que la guerra de sitios, cuyo efecto es el de hacer morir de hambre tanto a civiles como a combatientes.[12] El Convenio de La Haya de 1907 volvió a hacer hincapié en el principio de humanidad de la Cláusula de Martens y en el principio de necesidad.[13] Por lo tanto, la Convención de La Haya de 1907 podría ser interpretada como la prohibición de tácticas militares como el Plan del Hambre de los nazis, el cual utilizó el hambre como un medio para eliminar a los civiles en lugar de poner fin a la guerra.

Para tal efecto, el Tribunal Militar Internacional de Nuremberg (TMI-N) declaró en 1939 que las reglas de la guerra del Convenio de La Haya de 1907 pertenecían al derecho internacional consuetudinario:

> Las reglas de la guerra terrestre expresadas en la Convención (La Haya, 1907) representaban indudablemente un avance sobre el derecho internacional que existía al momento de su adop-

---

11. Rupert Ticehurst, "The Martens Clause and the Laws of Armed Conflict"[La cláusula de Martens y las leyes del conflicto armado], *International Review of the Red Cross* 317 (30 de abril de 1997), https://casebook.icrc.org/glossary/fundamental-prinaily-ihl; *Sin embargo, véase,* S. S. Lotus (Fr. v. Turk.), sentencia, 1927 P.C.I.J. Series A 16 No. 10 (7 de septiembre), pág. 19 (en su dicta, la Corte describe lo que se conoce como el segundo Principio de Loto, el cual sugiere crudamente que todo lo que no esté prohibido de manera expresa por el derecho internacional, está permitido: "Sin embargo, no se desprende que el derecho internacional prohíba a un Estado ejercer su jurisdicción en su propio territorio respecto de cualquier caso que se refiera a actos que hayan tenido lugar en el extranjero y en los que no pueda invocar alguna norma permisiva de derecho internacional. Esa opinión sólo sería sostenible si el derecho internacional incluyera una prohibición general a los Estados para hacer extensiva la aplicación de sus leyes y la jurisdicción de sus tribunales a las personas, los bienes y los actos 'fuera de su territorio'...").

12. El artículo 27 del Convenio IV de La Haya prohíbe a los beligerantes atacar a los enfermos y heridos durante el sitio de guerra, pero no específicamente a los civiles, y el artículo 28 prohíbe el saqueo de una ciudad o aldea sitiada. *Véase* Convenio (IV) relativo a las leyes y costumbres de la guerra terrestre y su anexo: Reglamento relativo a las leyes y costumbres de la guerra terrestre. La Haya, 18 de octubre de 1907; 27-28 [en lo sucesivo, Convenio IV de La Haya].

13. *Id*. en el Preámbulo.

ción...sin embargo, en 1939 estas reglas...fueron avaladas por
todas las naciones civilizadas y consideradas como una declara-
toria de las leyes y costumbres de la guerra.[14]

Sin embargo, a pesar de que la Convención de La Haya de 1907 prohíbe
a los beligerantes causar sufrimientos innecesarios y destruir bienes,[15] el
TMI-N no juzgó a los perpetradores nazis por el delito de provocación del
hambre como consecuencia del Plan del Hambre. Sin embargo, el TMI-N
acusó al General del Ejército Wilhelm von Leeb por el Sitio de Leningrado
en el juicio del Alto Mando. Como el nombre lo indica, el juicio del Alto
Mando fue el enjuiciamiento de doce altos oficiales nazis por sus presuntos
crímenes de guerra y crímenes contra la paz cometidos durante la Segunda
Guerra Mundial; el juicio de von Leeb tuvo lugar por el papel que este
desempeñó durante la invasión de la Unión Soviética durante la Operación
Barbarroja. El TMI-N determinó finalmente que, aunque el hambre como
consecuencia del sitio había sido atroz, no obstante, era legal:

> Un comandante beligerante puede sitiar legalmente un lugar
> controlado por el enemigo y procurar un proceso de aislamiento
> para provocar su rendición. La respetabilidad del intento para
> acelerarlo por medio del hambre no se cuestiona. Se dice que, si
> un comandante de un lugar sitiado expulsa a los no combatientes
> con el fin de reducir el número de consumidores de su inventario
> de provisiones, *es lícito, a pesar de ser una medida extrema, para
> forzarlos a retroceder si se expedita su rendición*...Por ende, la inter-
> rupción de toda fuente de sustento desde el exterior se considera
> legítimo...*Podríamos desear que la ley fuera diferente, pero debemos
> aplicarla tal como es*. En consecuencia, no existe criminalidad en
> conexión con este delito.[16]

De hecho, la práctica del estado sugería que las principales Partes en la
Segunda Guerra Mundial, con excepción de la Unión Soviética, creían que
el hambre con el fin de hacer capitular al enemigo era un método legítimo y
legal de guerra. Por ejemplo, los Estados Unidos y el Reino Unido recurrieron
al bloqueo de los suministros de alimentos de Alemania, el territorio ocupado

---

14. Tribunal Militar Internacional de Nuremberg, reimpreso en *AJIL* 41,248–249 (1947).
15. Convenio IV de La Haya, nota *supra* 12, en Art. 23.
16. Juicio de los Criminales de Guerra ante el Tribunal Militar de Núremberg según la
Ley Núm. 10 del Consejo de Control, octubre de 1946–abril de 1949, Vol. XI, 563 (U.S.
Government Printing Office, Washington, D.C., 1950) (énfasis añadido).

por Alemania y Japón; Estados Unidos incluso llamó a su bloqueo de puertos japoneses "Operación hambruna".[17] Así pues, el hambre provocada por los sitios y bloqueos realizados durante la Segunda Guerra Mundial no estaba prohibida de *ipso facto* por el derecho internacional. Sin embargo, aunque el hambre no estaba estrictamente prohibida durante la Segunda Guerra Mundial, eso no establece que el uso del hambre durante la guerra cumpliera con los principios de necesidad militar, proporcionalidad, distinción o humanidad.

Los horrores de la Segunda Guerra Mundial llevaron a dos acontecimientos importantes con respecto al derecho internacional: la Convención para la Prevención y la Sanción del Delito de Genocidio, de 1948, y el Convenio de Ginebra relativo a la Protección de las Personas Civiles, de 1949, los cuales prohíben expresamente el hacer padecer hambre a los civiles.[18] La Convención del Genocidio prohíbe "El sometimiento deliberado del grupo a condiciones de vida calculadas para llevar a la destrucción física, total o parcial".[19] Indudablemente, el hambre cumple con este criterio. En fechas más recientes en el año de 1977, los Protocolos Adicionales a las Convenios de Ginebra establecen una explicación detallada de los permisos y las prohibiciones sobre sitios, bloqueos, ataques contra los bienes indispensables para la supervivencia (BIS) y contra la ayuda humanitaria;[20] y el Estatuto de Roma de 1998[21] y las Enmiendas de 2019 penalizan el hambre como método de guerra tanto durante los conflictos armados internacionales sin carácter internacional.[22] Específicamente, el artículo 54 del Protocolo Adicional I y el artículo 14 del Protocolo Adicional II prohíben los ataques contra los bienes indispensables para la supervivencia y el hambre en los

---

17. Alex De Waal, *Mass Starvation: The History and Future of Famine* [El hambre masiva: historia y futuro de la hambruna] (2018), 127–28.

18. Convención para la Prevención y la Sanción del Delito de Genocidio, 9 de diciembre de 1948, 78 U.N.T.S. 277, Art. II(c); Convenio de Ginebra relativo a la protección de las personas civiles en tiempo de guerra, Ginebra, 8 de diciembre de 1949.

19. *Id*.

20. Protocolo adicional a los Convenios de Ginebra del 12 de agosto de 1949 relativo a la protección de las víctimas de los conflictos armados internacionales (Protocolo I), 8 de junio de 1977, 1125 U.N.T.S. 3, en Art. 54 (1) [en lo sucesivo, Protocolo I]; Protocolo adicional a los Convenios de Ginebra del 12 de agosto de 1949 relativo a la protección de las víctimas de los conflictos armados sin carácter internacional, 8 de junio de 1977, 1125 U.N.T.S. 609, en Arts. 14, 69-70 [en lo sucesivo, Protocolo II].

21. Estatuto de Roma de la Corte Penal Internacional, Art. 8(2)(b)(xxv), 17 de julio de 1998, UN Doc. A/CONF. 183/9, 2187 U.N.T.S. 9 [en lo sucesivo, Estatuto de Roma].

22. Asamblea de los Estados Parte de la Corte Penal Internacional, Informe del grupo de trabajo sobre las enmiendas, 18vo período de sesiones, 2–7 de diciembre de 2019, 7–9, ICC-ASP/18/32 (3 de diciembre de 2019), https://asp.icc-cpi.int/iccdocs/asp_docs/ASP18/ICC-ASP-18-32-ENG.pdf.

civiles, mientras que el artículo 70 del Protocolo Adicional I exige el flujo sin restricciones de la ayuda humanitaria.[23] Si bien el hambre en las personas civiles queda estrictamente prohibida conforme al Artículo 54, los sitios y bloqueos constituyen excepciones lícitas a las prohibiciones del hambre siempre que el ataque cumpla con los principios de necesidad militar, distinción y proporcionalidad, y no prive a los civiles de alimentos o agua adecuados, ni los obligue a retirarse por falta de los mismos.[24] Por último, el Estatuto de Roma de la Corte Penal Internacional (CPI) tipifica el hambre como un crimen de guerra cuando el perpetrador tiene la intención de provocar hambre en las personas civiles como método de guerra, los priva de los bienes indispensables para la supervivencia u obstaculiza intencionalmente los suministros de socorro.[25]

Aunque la ley ha evolucionado para imponer mayores restricciones sobre los métodos de guerra que provoquen el hambre, hoy en día el DIH, el DIP y el derecho internacional consuetudinario se quedan cortos en cuanto a la prohibición absoluta del uso del hambre como un arma de guerra. Por lo tanto, cualquier cambio en la ley debe ser producto de un desarrollo progresivo. Como expongo a continuación, por tratarse de un *malum in se* conforme al derecho internacional, el hambre debería estar totalmente prohibida. Asimismo, aplicaré el Principio del Doble Efecto (PDE) en algunos de los siguientes argumentos. El PDE es un ejercicio filosófico que explica la permisibilidad de una acción dañina, como el hambre en los civiles, o el resultado de promover alguna buena intención, como el terminar una guerra prolongada. Para que una acción sea moralmente permisible conforme al PDE, deben reunirse cuatro condiciones:

1. La acción debe ser moralmente buena o moralmente indiferente;
2. La intención del agente debe ser la de lograr un buen efecto y no uno malo. Si el agente puede lograr el buen efecto sin el malo, eso es entonces lo que se requiere;

---

23. Protocolo I, nota *supra* 20, en arts. 54(1) y 70; Protocolo II, nota *supra* 20, en el Art. 14.
24. *Id.* en el Protocolo Adicional I, art. 54(3).
25. Estatuto de Roma, nota *supra* 21, at art. 8(2)(b)(xxv)("Intentionally using starvation as a method of warfare by depriving civilians of objects indispensable to their survival, including willfully impeding relief supplies as provided for under the Geneva Conventions."["Utilizar intencionalmente el hambre como método de guerra privando a los civiles de los bienes indispensables para la supervivencia, incluso obstaculizando de manera intencional, los suministros de socorro de conformidad con los Convenios de Ginebra"]; *Véase también* Elements of Crimes [Elementos de los crímenes], Corte Penal Internacional (2001), en el art. 8 (2)(b)(xxv), https://www.icc-cpi.int/nr/rdonlyres/336923d8-a6ad-40ec-ad7b-45bf9de73d56/0/elementsofcrimeseng.pdf.

3. El buen efecto debe producirse directamente como resultado de la acción, y no por el mal efecto (por ejemplo, no se permite usar un mal medio para lograr un buen fin);

4. El buen efecto debe ser lo suficientemente deseable como para compensar el permitir el mal efecto (por ejemplo, el bien logrado debe ser proporcional al mal permitido).[26]

Una campaña de hambre no cumple claramente con la primera condición, ya que el hambre nunca puede ser moralmente bueno o moralmente indiferente. Incluso si la táctica de un bloqueo pudiera considerarse como moralmente indiferente, si el efecto del bloqueo es el de provocar hambre, entonces el bloqueo no cumple con la tercera condición puesto que un mal efecto (el hambre, por ejemplo) nunca debe ser usado para lograr un buen fin (por ejemplo, el de evitar que las armas lleguen a manos enemigas).

Parte II: La utilización del hambre como arma de guerra es *malum in se*

La utilización del hambre como método de guerra constituye un acto *malum in se* puesto que viola los principios *jus in bello* de distinción, proporcionalidad, necesidad y daño superfluo.

El hambre como arma de guerra viola el principio de distinción del *jus in bello*.

El hambre, por naturaleza, es un arma indiscriminada. El DIH exige que los ataques militares distingan entre los civiles y los combatientes. Cuando el hambre se utiliza lícitamente, ya sea mediante el sitio o el bloqueo, es imposible distinguir entre civiles y combatientes. Es por ello que los Protocolos Adicionales requieren que los combatientes (1) permitan que la ayuda humanitaria se distribuya entre los civiles durante los bloqueos y sitios y/o (2) permitan que los civiles salgan de las ciudades sitiadas. Del mismo modo, cualquier otro ataque al territorio enemigo, por lo demás legítimo, puede provocar hambre si este destruye los bienes necesarios para la supervivencia. Como los suministros de agua y los emplazamientos agrícolas son aprovechados tanto por civiles como por combatientes, la destrucción de los bienes necesarios para la supervivencia destinados a forzar la capitulación del enemigo es *malum in se,* puesto que dichos ataques son indiscriminados.

Hay quienes podrían argumentar que cuando su uso es lícito, el hambre provocada por sitios, bloqueos o ataques en perjuicio de los bienes necesarios para la supervivencia dirigidos a los combatientes no es *malum in se* siempre

---

26. Stephen Coleman, *Military Ethics: An Introduction with Case Studies* [Ética militar: una introducción con casos de estudio] (Oxford University Press 2012), 22.

y cuando se limite el sufrimiento civil. Hasta ese punto, el problema no es que los sitios, los bloqueos o los ataques contra los bienes necesarios para la supervivencia no puedan distinguir entre civiles y combatientes, sino más bien, que los combatientes opten por no hacer dicha distinción. Estos malos actores violan así el DCA y deben ser castigados de conformidad con los Convenios de Ginebra o el Estatuto de Roma.

La realidad, sin embargo, es que incluso los combatientes "bien" intencionados que sitian, bloquean o atacan no pueden garantizar del todo, que estas tácticas no harán daño a los civiles. De esta manera, los métodos de guerra que provocan el hambre no satisfacen la cuarta condición del PDE, a saber, que el "buen" efecto de propiciar la capitulación del enemigo no es lo suficientemente deseable como para compensar que se permita el mal efecto de hacer padecer hambre a los civiles de forma indiscriminada. Además, en muchos casos, si no en su mayoría, la ayuda humanitaria no llega a los civiles ya sea por el pillaje de los beligerantes o porque es destruida en su trayecto hacia los civiles. Y los civiles no siempre son capaces de abandonar las ciudades sitiadas. Los ancianos, los discapacitados y los niños pequeños, hacia quienes existe una responsabilidad especial de cuidados tanto legales como éticos, no pueden trasladarse fácilmente y a menudo no tienen a donde ir. Por lo tanto, incluso con la mejor de las intenciones, los civiles sufren un daño enorme cuando los sitios, bloqueos y ataques contra los bienes indispensables para la supervivencia son utilizados como un método de guerra. Lo anterior se evidencia en los numerosos casos de hambruna durante los conflictos armados de los últimos cien años, pero especialmente en los recientes conflictos en Sudán, Siria y Yemen, donde cientos de miles de civiles han muerto a causa del hambre y de enfermedades vinculadas con la guerra.[27]

El hambre como arma de guerra viola el principio de proporcionalidad del *jus in bello.*

El hambre se traduce a menudo en muertes desproporcionadas. El principio de proporcionalidad del *jus in bello* prohíbe a los combatientes lanzar un ataque o utilizar medios de guerra que *puedan* ocasionar daños extremos a la población civil. Independientemente de si los sitios, bloqueos o ataques contra los bienes indispensables para la supervivencia son legales, con frecuencia producen exceso de daños a la población civil. El Plan del Hambre de los

---

27. *Véase* Jennifer Trahan, *Existing Legal Limits to Security Council Veto Power in the Face of Atrocity Crimes* [Límites legales existentes del poder del veto del Consejo de Seguridad frente a crímenes atroces],278–79 (Cambridge University Press 2020); *véase también*, Laura Graham, "Pathways to Accountability for Starvation Crimes in Yemen", *[Vías hacia la rendición de cuentas por los delitos de hambre en Yemen]* Case Western J. of Intl. L. 53 (2020).

nazis provocó la muerte de más de cuatro millones de personas,[28] y la actual guerra civil en Yemen ha puesto a trece millones de personas en riesgo de muerte o desnutrición aguda y enfermedad derivadas del hambre.[29] En el contexto del Plan del Hambre, donde los nazis planeaban alimentar al ejército alemán mediante el pillaje de alimentos en la Unión Soviética, la muerte de hambre de 4.7 millones de personas no es ni proporcional a un objetivo militar legítimo ni se justifica bajo la segunda condición del PDE, en la cual el agente debe tener la intención de lograr el buen efecto con la acción, y no uno malo. Los nazis no pretendían lograr un buen efecto. Como mostraré en el caso de estudio en la tercera parte de este ensayo, mientras que uno de los propósitos del Plan del Hambre (alimentar al ejército alemán) podría ser considerado como legítimo si se cumplieran otras condiciones, el propósito principal era el de exterminar a los soviéticos. El exterminio de un grupo nacional o étnico es un genocidio, el cual siempre es *malum in se*. Y con respecto a los trece millones de personas en riesgo de muerte por la hambruna en Yemen debido a bloqueos y ataques contra los bienes indispensables para la supervivencia, incluso si se persiguiera un objetivo militar legítimo con estas tácticas, la enorme cantidad de civiles en riesgo de muerte y enfermedades (aproximadamente el 45 por ciento de la población)[30] es excesivo y, por lo tanto, no es proporcional a un objetivo militar legítimo.

Un contraargumento respecto a la opinión de que la utilización del hambre como método de guerra es desproporcionada es aquel que cuando se utiliza el hambre para expeditar la capitulación del enemigo puede, en última instancia, salvar vidas inocentes. Con ese fin, muchos historiadores de guerra consideran que la utilización del hambre en contra de los alemanes durante la Primera y la Segunda Guerra Mundial intensificó su capitulación, salvando a un sinnúmero de vidas.[31] Hay quienes podrían argumentar que si dichas tácticas propician la capitulación del enemigo más rápido en comparación con una campaña militar sostenida, entonces debiéramos tomar en cuenta las bajas civiles de sitios, bloqueos y destrucción de los bienes indispensables para la supervivencia como proporcionales a lo que hubiera sido una mayor pérdida de vidas durante un conflicto prolongado.

---

28. De Waal, nota *supra* 17, en 104
29. BBC News, "Yemen could be 'worst famine in 100 years,'" ["Yemen podría ser 'la peor hambruna en 100 años'"] (15 de octubre de 2018), https://www.bbc.com/news/av/world-middle-east-45857729.
30. Banco Mundial, "Total Population Yemen" [Población total de Yemen], https://data.worldbank.org/indicator/SP.POP.TOTL?locations=YE.
31. *Véase, en general,* Lizzie Collingham, *The Taste of War: World War II and the Battle for Food* (2012).[El sabor de la guerra: la Segunda Guerra Mundial y la lucha por los alimentos]

Sin embargo, para entender mejor la pérdida de vidas debido a la hambruna en la Primera y la Segunda Guerras Mundiales, debe ampliarse el período de tiempo. La pérdida de vidas civiles no ocurre sólo durante los días o meses contiguos a un sitio o bloqueo; más bien, la pérdida de vidas debe calcularse a lo largo de meses y en ocasiones, de años de inseguridad alimentaria y enfermedades provocadas por el sitio o bloqueo, incluso después de terminarse la guerra. En Alemania, "el invierno de los nabos", de 1916 a 1917, provocado en parte por los embargos estadounidenses, representó la muerte de por lo menos 750 mil alemanes a causa de la desnutrición y la tasa de natalidad cayó de forma considerable.[32] Muchas de esas muertes ocurrieron durante los seis meses *posteriores* al armisticio.[33] Durante la Segunda Guerra Mundial, al menos veinte millones de personas murieron de hambre, desnutrición y enfermedades relacionadas con la misma.[34] De esos veinte millones, un millón murió durante el Sitio de Leningrado.[35] En ese contexto, está claro que la pérdida de vidas civiles es mucho mayor de lo que se permitiría en virtud del principio de proporcionalidad.

El hambre como arma de guerra viola el principio de necesidad del *jus in bello.*

El hambre nunca es necesaria en la guerra. El principio de necesidad del *jus in bello* permite la adopción de medidas *realmente* necesarias para lograr un propósito militar legítimo. Impedir que las armas y otros suministros lleguen a manos enemigas es un propósito militar legítimo que puede lograrse mediante un bloqueo. Sin embargo, cuando los bloqueos también impiden que la ayuda humanitaria llegue a los civiles o se les permita tener acceso a alimentos o agua, esos métodos de guerra son moralmente inadmisibles puesto que provocan sufrimientos y daños innecesarios a los civiles. Y como un propósito militar legítimo no puede conseguirse éticamente a través de medios que sean moralmente corruptos, el hambre, independientemente de que sea una consecuencia directa o indirecta de un método lícito de guerra, no satisfará el principio de necesidad.

Los opositores a la prohibición absoluta de los sitios, bloqueos y otros métodos lícitos de guerra que emplean la táctica del hambre consideran que tales prohibiciones eliminarían un arma vital que los militares *podrían* necesitar en ciertos casos excepcionales. Por ejemplo, cuando la derrota militar es inevitable, *excepto* cuando se sitia un bastión enemigo-combatiente o un bloqueo para evitar el flujo de municiones hacia el enemigo, estos

---

32. *Id*. en 25.
33. De Waal, nota *supra* 17, en 74
34. Collingham, nota *supra* 31, en 2
35. *Id*. en 5.

medios de guerra pudieran ser entonces, una necesidad *real*. A diferencia de la violación o el genocidio, que son *mala in se* puesto que *nunca* se justifican,[36] los opositores podrían argumentar que, en ciertos casos excepcionales, como en una "emergencia suprema",[37]el hambre no solo es el menor de los males, sino que también se justifica para evitar una tragedia peor o la derrota. Y cuando las necesidades legítimas de un objetivo militar superan de manera considerable, al número de muertes civiles a causa del hambre, se justifica su uso bajo el principio de necesidad.

Si bien pueden presentarse emergencias supremas excepcionales que justifiquen el tomar medidas extremas para evitar la aniquilación humana, en el mundo real, siempre habrá alguna alternativa al uso de sitios, bloqueos y ataques contra los bienes indispensables para la supervivencia. Bajo la segunda condición del PDE, no se justifica la acción si el agente puede lograr el buen efecto (la victoria militar) sin el mal efecto (el hambre). Además, en el análisis de Orend, el concepto de Walzer sobre una emergencia suprema corrompe la tradición de la Guerra Justa al descartar las justificaciones morales de los requisitos del *jus in bello*.[38] Siguiendo esta lógica, el hambre como método de guerra nunca podría ser justificado, ni siquiera en caso de emergencia suprema puesto que permitir un acto tan vil corrompería los fundamentos morales de los principios del *jus in bello*. Por lo tanto, aunque el hambre sea un método eficiente para llevar al enemigo a la capitulación, no es una necesidad militar real, ni siquiera en circunstancias extremas. Incluso si el hambre como método de guerra fuera *realmente* necesaria debido a una amenaza existencial, el sufrimiento ocasionado por tal método es vil en sí mismo y debe prohibirse totalmente. Por lo tanto, el argumento de la necesidad suprema en caso de emergencia no es convincente puesto que el hacer padecer hambre a personas inocentes es sustancialmente vil y nunca puede justificarse conforme a los requisitos del *jus in bello*.[39]

El hambre como arma de guerra viola el principio de daño superficial del *jus in bello*.

El hambre ocasiona daños superfluos o innecesarios tanto en los civiles como en los combatientes. Al igual que las minas terrestres, las municiones

---

36. *Véase* Morten Dige, *Explaining the Principle of Mala in Se* [Explicando el principio de *mala in se*], *J. Mil. Ethics* 11(2012), 318–332, 319.
37. Michael Walzer, *Just and Unjust Wars* [Guerras justas e injustas], 252 (1977).
38. Brian Orend, *The Morality of War* [La moralidad de la guerra], 147–148 (2006); *Véase también*, Martin Cook, "Michael Walzer 's Concept of 'Supreme Emergency '", [El concepto de Michael Walzer sobre la 'emergencia suprema']*J. Mil. Ethics* 6 [Ética 6] (2007):138–151, 143.
39. *Véase, por ejemplo*, Dige, nota *supra* 36, en 319.

en racimo, las armas biológicas y demás armas que son ilegales debido a sus efectos perniciosos, el hambre como herramienta de guerra es insidiosa. La muerte provocada por el hambre es un proceso agonizante. Al ser humano promedio le toma dos meses completos para morir de hambre[40] Según Lizzie Collingham, experta en alimentos y guerra:

> Las víctimas de la hambruna mueren por distrofia nutricional, un proceso por el cual, una vez que el cuerpo ha agotado todas sus reservas de grasa, los músculos se descomponen para obtener energía. El intestino delgado se atrofia y cada vez es más difícil para la víctima la absorción de nutrientes de los pocos alimentos que pudiera obtener. Como mecanismo de defensa, el cuerpo disminuye la actividad de los órganos vitales como el corazón y el hígado, y la víctima sufre, no sólo de debilidad muscular, sino de una fatiga más general y abrumadora…El volumen de agua en el cuerpo se reduce a un ritmo más lento que el del desgaste de los músculos y tejidos y aumenta la flacidez del cuerpo. Algunas víctimas de la hambruna desarrollan edemas debido al hambre y se hinchan con el excedente de agua. La hinchazón comienza en el abdomen y en las piernas y se extiende por todo el cuerpo. La piel se vuelve estirada, brillante e hipersensible. La presión arterial disminuye y la víctima se plaga de queratitis (enrojecimiento y dolor de la córnea), dolor de las encías, dolores de cabeza, dolores en las piernas, dolores neurálgicos, temblores y ataxia (pérdida de control sobre las extremidades). Los síntomas van acompañados de un antojo intenso de carbohidratos y sal, y se presenta una diarrea incontrolable. Justo antes de la muerte, la víctima cambia bruscamente de la depresión a la irritación intensa y luego se sumerge en un profundo letargo. Al final, el cuerpo no tiene otra alternativa que la de mantenerse vivo tomando proteínas de los órganos vitales…Lo que es más importante, el corazón se atrofia…La insuficiencia orgánica es la causa final de la muerte.[41]

No existe ningún beneficio militar que pueda justificar el uso de esta perniciosa arma.

Hay quienes podrían argumentar que la humanidad ha utilizado el hambre como un arma de guerra durante milenios. Si fuera tan terrible,

---

40. De Waal, nota *supra* 17, en 21.
41. Collingham, nota *supra* 31, en 5-6.

no se permitiría más durante las guerras y se enjuiciaría a los autores de crímenes de hambre provocada. Entre otras cosas, nunca se ha castigado a nadie por los crímenes relacionados con el hambre. La falta de prohibiciones y procesos judiciales pueden evidenciar que la comunidad internacional considera aceptable el uso de esta táctica o al menos más aceptable que la de las minas terrestres, municiones en racimo y las armas biológicas. Además, podría argumentarse que las muertes de combatientes a causa del hambre no son peores que las provocadas por los bombardeos y demás medios legales de la guerra. De hecho, debido a que el propósito específico de los sitios y bloqueos no es el de matar de hambre al enemigo, sino el de hacer que se someta y se rinda, los efectos perniciosos del hambre en las últimas fases de la insuficiencia orgánica es un suceso poco probable puesto que el enemigo seguramente capitulará mucho antes de entrar en esa fase.

Sin embargo, este argumento fracasa debido a que la falta de enjuiciamiento de los autores de los crímenes del hambre constituye un problema de voluntad política y un estancamiento en el Consejo de Seguridad de la ONU y no un reflejo de la falta de percepción internacional en cuanto al horror que el hambre conlleva. El hecho de que la comunidad internacional no haya tomado las medidas necesarias para poner fin a los bloqueos y ataques contra los bienes indispensables para la supervivencia en Yemen, por ejemplo, no significa que no se haya hecho el esfuerzo. El Consejo de Seguridad de la ONU aprobó la Resolución 2417, en un esfuerzo por condenar el hambre como resultado de la guerra en Yemen, y una enmienda al Estatuto de Roma en el año 2019 que amplía el concepto del hambre como crimen de guerra y su ejecución en conflictos armados sin carácter internacional.[42] La escasez de enjuiciamientos relativos a los crímenes del hambre simplemente refleja la geopolítica de nuestro orden internacional actual. Si bien es posible que haya intentos fallidos para salvar a Yemen, a largo plazo, la balanza de la justicia se va inclinando hacia la imposición de prohibiciones más estrictas, y quizá absolutas, con respecto al hambre como método de guerra. Además, la idea de que el enemigo capitulará antes de que se sientan los efectos perniciosos del hambre, no está respaldada por ninguna evidencia histórica. De hecho, lo que tiende a ocurrir durante los sitios y bloqueos es que los combatientes enemigos reserven raciones

---

42. S.C. Res. 2417, ¶¶ 5–7 (24 de mayo de 2018); Asamblea de los Estados Partes de la Corte Penal Internacional, Informe del Grupo de Trabajo sobre las Enmiendas, decimoctavo período de sesiones, del 2–7 de diciembre de 2019, 7–9, ICC-ASP/18/32 (3 de diciembre de 2019), https://asp.icc-cpi.int/iccdocs/asp_docs/ASP18/ICC-ASP-18-32-ENG.pdf.

de alimentos vitales y agua para sí mismos, lo que exacerba la precariedad de los civiles en las zonas de guerra. De hecho, son los civiles los que más sufren durante los sitios y bloqueos debido a las cantidades limitadas de alimentos o agua, a la falta de acceso a agua potable y porque, con frecuencia, los civiles son personas ya sea muy jóvenes, de edad avanzada, enfermas o mujeres embarazadas, todos los cuales tienen menores probabilidades de poder soportar la escasez de alimentos por un período de tiempo prolongado. Independientemente de si son muchos o pocos los que mueren de hambre, el principio del daño superfluo prohíbe infligir sufrimiento innecesario, y la muerte por hambre es una forma intolerablemente cruel de morir.

Parte III: Casos de estudio relacionados con el hambre: El Plan del hambre de los nazis y la guerra civil en Yemen

El plan del hambre de los nazis

Está bien establecido que los alemanes capitularon en la Primera Guerra Mundial porque estaban hambrientos y ya no podían llevar a cabo sus objetivos militares sin el acceso a suministros adecuados de alimentos.[43] Cerca de 750 mil ciudadanos alemanes murieron como resultado de la desnutrición derivada de la guerra.[44] En el período previo a la Segunda Guerra Mundial, el hecho de que tantos alemanes hubieran padecido hambre durante la Primera Guerra Mundial estaba muy a la vanguardia de las preocupaciones y planes que tenía Hitler para el dominio mundial.[45] Debido a una combinación de no querer que se repitiera la derrota de Alemania, como ocurrió durante la Primera Guerra Mundial, y al plan nazi para la expansión del espacio habitado por los alemanes, gracias a la política de Lebensraum, los nazis confiaron en el Ministerio del Reich para la Alimentación y la Agricultura para que desarrollara políticas que abordaran la escasez de alimentos y el racionamiento para ayudar a que los nazis lograran la victoria durante la guerra.[46] Si bien gran parte del trabajo del Ministerio durante la primera parte de la guerra fue el de incrementar la producción de alimentos en Alemania y en los territorios de ocupación nazi, así como racionar los alimentos destinados a los civiles y soldados alemanes, el Ministerio también fue el

---

43. *Id. Véase también* Alex De Waal, nota *supra* 17, en 74; Gesine Gerhard, "Food and Genocide: Nazi Agrarian Politics in the Occupied Territories of the Soviet Union" [Alimentos y genocidio: la política agraria en los territorios ocupados por la Unión Soviética], *Contemporary European History* 18, 45 -65.

44. De Waal, nota *supra* 17.

45. *Id.* en 75.

46. *Id.* en 101.

responsable de establecer los requerimientos calóricos para las víctimas del holocausto en los campos de concentración así como de los prisioneros de guerra.[47] A las víctimas de los nazis se les permitía consumir tan solo entre 184 y 845 calorías diarias, o sea, una dieta de hambre.[48]

Para el año 1941, estaba claro que para que los nazis derrotaran al Ejército Rojo y buscaran el dominio global, el Wehrmacht (el ejército alemán) necesitaría de un suministro continuo de alimentos, del que no se disponía en Alemania.[49] Los nazis calcularon que cada uno de los 9.5 millones de hombres del ejército tendría que consumir 3,000 calorías diarias para realizar las actividades militares.[50] En 1943, el Wehrmacht consumía el 40% del total de los granos y el 62% del total de la carne disponible para el Reich, provocando la escasez de alimentos disponibles para los civiles en Alemania.[51] El arma más valiosa de la guerra era, por lo tanto, los alimentos.

Temiendo que se repitiera la derrota de Alemania como ocurrió durante la Primera Guerra Mundial, los nazis desarrollaron un plan que los ayudaría a derrotar al Ejército Rojo y a suministrar alimentos suficientes para los alemanes por el tiempo que durara la guerra.[52] Entre marzo y mayo de 1941, tuvo lugar una serie de reuniones de alto nivel entre Herbert Backe, el autor del Plan del Hambre; Hermann Göring, Plenipotenciario del Plan Cuatrienal y Comandante Supremo de la Luftwaffe (Fuerza Aérea); Adolf Hitler; y otros líderes nazis de alto rango, en relación con el Plan Cuatrienal del Partido Nazi para la victoria.[53] El resultado de esas reuniones fue un plan para matar de hambre a treinta millones de "bocas inútiles" en la Unión Soviética.[54] El Plan del Hambre identificó zonas con excedente de producción de alimentos y zonas deficitarias en la Unión Soviética.[55] Las zonas excedentarias, principalmente en Ucrania, conocida como el granero de la Unión Soviética, así como el sur de Rusia y la región del Cáucaso, serían captadas por el Wehrmacht y utilizadas para enviar 8.7 millones de toneladas de excedentes de alimentos a Alemania, mientras que a las zonas deficitarias, o sea, los grandes centros

---

47. Collingham, nota *supra* 31, en 4–5.
48. *Id.*
49. *Id.* en 179–180.
50. *Id.* en 180.
51. *Id.*
52. De Waal, nota *supra* 17, at 102; Gerhard, nota *supra* 43, en 46–47.
53. Alex J. Kay, *Exploitation, Resettlement, Mass Murder: Political and Economic Planning for German Occupation Policy in the Soviet Union* [Explotación, reasentamiento, asesinato en masa: planificación política y económica para la política de ocupación alemana en la Unión Soviética], *1940–1941*, 47–67 (2011 e-book).
54. De Waal, nota *supra* 17, en 102; Gerhard, nota *supra* 43, en 46.
55. Gerhard, nota *supra* 43, en 56–57.

urbanos, como Moscú, en el norte y centro de Rusia, que requerían de alimentos, debía interrumpírseles todo el suministro de alimentos con el fin de exterminar a la población.[56] El resultado de la política, de haber tenido éxito, habría sumido en la hambruna a treinta millones de personas eslavas y judías de la Unión Soviética.[57]

En mayo de 1941, los nazis celebraron una conferencia en Wannsee, una pequeña ciudad lacustre situada a las afueras de Berlín. Después de la Conferencia de Wannsee, se distribuyó entre los altos funcionarios nazis un documento de veinte páginas sobre las Directrices de la Política Económica para la Organización Económica del Este en el que se esbozaba el Plan del Hambre.[58] El documento señalaba:

> La población de estos territorios, en particular la población de las ciudades tendrá que enfrentarse a la hambruna más terrible…Muchas decenas de millones de personas en este territorio se volverán innecesarias y morirán o deberán emigrar a Siberia. Los intentos por reducir en esa área el nivel de la población por medio del hambre provocada, reteniendo los excedentes de la zona de tierra negra, sólo son viables a costa del suministro de Europa. Estas personas evitan la posibilidad de que Alemania resista hasta el fin de la guerra, impiden que Alemania y Europa resistan el bloqueo.[59]

Los nazis formalizaron su plan de hambre y luego instigaron el peor crimen del hambre de la historia.[60]

Los nazis siguieron adelante con el Plan del Hambre encubierto bajo la Operación Barbarroja, o sea, la invasión de los países del Eje a la Unión Soviética.[61] Pero calcularon mal el peso de la ofensiva y, al final, no pudieron lograr la victoria contra el Ejército Rojo debido a la deserción, es decir, el Ejército Rojo había derrotado al Wehrmacht gracias a la pérdida continua de soldados.[62] Los nazis subestimaron seriamente la dificultad de derrotar al

---

56. *Id. Véase también* Kay, nota *supra* 53, en 127.
57. De Waal, nota *supra* 17, en 102-3.
58. Gerhard, nota *supra* 43, en 58.
59. Kay, nota *supra* 53, en 135.
60. De Waal, nota *supra* 17, en 15.
61. *Id.* en 102.
62. Holocaust Encyclopedia, "Invasion of the Soviet Union, June 1941, US Holocaust Memorial Museum" [Invasión de la Unión Soviética, junio de 1941, Museo Conmemorativo del Holocausto de EE. UU."], https://encyclopedia.ushmm.org/content/en/article/invasion-of-thesoviet-union-june-1941.

Ejército Rojo, el cual superaba en número al Wehrmacht en una proporción de 2:1.[63] A pesar de calcular erróneamente la fuerza del Ejército Rojo, los nazis lograron una pequeña parte de su propósito, previsto en el Plan del Hambre; la Operación Barbarroja significó la muerte de un millón de soviéticos debido a la hambruna por el período de novecientos días que durara el Sitio de Leningrado.[64] Alrededor de uno o dos millones de prisioneros de guerra soviéticos murieron de hambre en los campos de trabajos forzados de los nazis.[65]

Una de las principales razones por las que el Plan del Hambre fracasó en cuanto a su objetivo principal, fue debido a que los nazis subestimaron la dificultad y el tiempo necesario para matar de hambre a treinta millones de personas. Para que el ser humano promedio muera de hambre debe pasar dos meses sin alimentos.[66] Por ejemplo, Bobby Sands, el huelguista de hambre del Ejército Republicano Irlandés (IRA, por sus siglas en inglés), murió por falta de alimentos luego de sesenta y seis días.[67] Pero los nazis nunca fueron capaces de interrumpir por completo el suministro de alimentos a la Unión Soviética, lo que se debió, en parte, a la disponibilidad de alimentos en el mercado negro.[68] Y así tomó mucho más tiempo matar de hambre a la población, todo mientras trataban de derrotar al Ejército Rojo por medio del combate. Era demasiado ambicioso para lograrlo y, finalmente los nazis se retiraron.[69] El Plan del Hambre de los nazis, que planeaba dar muerte a treinta millones de personas, terminó al final, matando a cerca de 4.7 millones.[70] De haber tenido éxito, hubiera significado la peor atrocidad jamás cometida.

A pesar del hecho de que 4.7 millones de personas murieron de hambre bajo el Plan del Hambre, ni Herbert Backe, ni Hermann Göring, ni Walter Darré, quien fuera el Ministro del Reich para la Alimentación y la Agricultura durante el Plan del Hambre, fueron juzgados por haber violado las leyes de

---

63. Reina Pennington, "Was the Russian Military a Steamroller? From World War II to Today" [¿Era el ejécito rojo una aplanadora? De la Segunda Guerra Mundial al presente], *War on the Rocks* (6 de julio de 2016), https://warontherocks.com/2016/07/was-the-russian-military-a-steamroller-from-world-war-ii-to-today/.

64. Collingham, nota *supra* 31, en 5.

65. *Id.* en 193; Gerhard, nota *supra* 43, en 60-61.

66. Collingham, nota *supra* 31, en 5-6; De Waal, nota *supra* 17, en 21.

67. *Id.*

68. Kay, nota *supra* 53, en 134-35.

69. Encyclopedia Britannica Online, "Stalingrad and the German retreat, summer 1942–February 1943," [Stanligrado y el retiro alemán, verano de 1942 a febrero de 1943] https://www.britannica.com/event/World-War-II/Stalingrad-and-the-German-retreat-summer-1942-February-1943.

70. De Waal, nota *supra* 17, en 104 (señalando que es imposible saber con exactitud a cuánto ascendió el número de muertos del Plan del Hambre, pero ajustándose a la cifra de 4.7 millones y basándose en los cálculos de los principales historiadores).

la guerra en relación con el hambre provocada en los civiles como método de guerra. Las razones tienen que ver con la costumbre de la época, en la que no se prohibía el hacer padecer hambre como un método de guerra. Sin embargo, como he argumentado anteriormente, la utilización del hambre como un arma del Plan del Hambre de los nazis es *malum in se* porque nunca puede ser justificada moral o éticamente conforme a los principios del DIH y porque no cumple con las cuatro condiciones del PDE. No cumple la primera condición porque el hambre utilizada como arma no es ni moralmente benéfica ni moralmente indiferente. No cumple con la segunda condición porque la intención de los nazis nunca fue la de producir un buen efecto, sino la de exterminar a 30 millones de soviéticos a la vez que se alimentaba al ejército alemán. La tercera condición no se cumple puesto que el hacer padecer hambre a más de cuatro millones de personas es un mal efecto que carece de justificación. Y la cuarta condición tampoco se cumple debido a que el discutible "buen" efecto de desviar alimentos de la Unión Soviética para alimentar al ejército alemán no puede compensar el mal efecto de matar de hambre a 4.7 millones de personas. Por lo tanto, el Plan del Hambre no se justifica de conformidad con los principios del DIH y ni cumple con el PDE.

La guerra civil en Yemen

La guerra en Yemen ha originado la peor crisis humanitaria del mundo.[71] Debido a la guerra civil en curso entre los rebeldes hutíes y el gobierno yemení, y que diera comienzo en 2015, el hambre y las enfermedades se han generalizado, dejando una estela de decenas de miles de muertes civiles. Más de veinte millones de personas padecen de inseguridad alimentaria y de enfermedades prevenibles como el cólera y la desnutrición aguda.[72]

---

71. Observaciones del Secretario General a la Conferencia de promesas de contribuciones en Yemen, Oficina de las Naciones Unidas en Ginebra (1ro de abril de 2018), https://www.unog.ch/unog/website/news_media.nsf/(httpNewsByYear_en)/27F6CCAD7178 F3E9C1258264003311FA?OpenDocument; *Véase también* Stephen O'Brien, Declaración ante el Consejo de Seguridad sobre Misiones en Yemen, Sudán del Sur, Somalia y Kenia y una actualización sobre la Conferencia de Oslo sobre Nigeria y la Región del Lago Chad, Consejo de Seguridad de las Naciones Unidas (10 de marzo de 2017) https://docs.unocha.org/sites/dms/Documents/ERC_USG_Stephen_OBrien_Statement_to_the_SecCo_on_Missions_to_Yemen_South_Sudan_Somalia_and_Kenya_and_update_on_Oslo.pdf (El jefe de la Oficina de las Naciones Unidas Stephen O'Brien dirigiéndose al Consejo de Seguridad "Estamos en un punto crítico de la historia. Desde principios de año nos enfrentamos a la mayor crisis humanitaria que ha habido desde la creación de las Naciones Unidas.") [en lo sucesivo, Declaración de O'Brien, 2017].
72. Humanitarian Aid, "Humanitarian crisis in Yemen remains the worst in the world, warns UN," [La crisis humanitaria en Yemen sigue siendo la peor del mundo, advierte la ONU] *UN News* (14 de febrero de 2019), https://news.un.org/en/

Desde el año 2017, se ha declarado que un estimado de trece millones de yemeníes están en riesgo de morir de hambre[73] y al menos 85 mil niños han muerto de hambre y de enfermedades relacionadas con la misma.[74] Yemen ha estado en la cuerda floja de la hambruna desde antes de que estallara la guerra en el año 2015.

Como la nación más pobre del Medio Oriente, aproximadamente el 44% de los yemeníes sufrían de desnutrición en el año 2012, y hasta cinco millones de personas dependían de la ayuda alimentaria de emergencia.[75] La escasez de agua era un problema de tal magnitud para este árido país que en el año 2012 los expertos predijeron que se agotaría toda el agua del país para el 2017.[76] A principios de ese mismo año, la ONU declaró a Yemen en peligro de hambruna inminente.[77] Una hambruna es "una crisis de hambre masiva que ocasiona una tasa de mortalidad elevada durante un período específico de tiempo"[78] y se debe a múltiples causas que incluyen "tanto a factores estructurales que determinan la vulnerabilidad como a detonantes inmediatos de la crisis".[79] Las hambrunas pueden distinguirse por su magnitud (el número de víctimas) y su gravedad (el nivel de inseguridad

---

story/2019/02/1032811; Doctors Without Borders/Médecins Sans Frontières (MSF) ha atendido 143,467 casos de cólera y 23,319 de desnutrición entre marzo de 2015 y septiembre de 2019. *Véase* Médecins Sans Frontières, "Yemen: Crisis Update November 2019", [Yemen: últimas noticias de la crisis de noviembre de 2019] https://www. doctorswithoutborders.org/what-we-do/news-stories/story/yemen-crisis-update-november-2019.

73. BBC News, "Yemen could be 'worst famine in 100 years,'" ["Yemen podría significar 'la peor hambruna en 100 años'"] (15 de octubre de 2018), https://www.bbc.com/news/av/world-middle-east-45857729.

74. Bethan McKernan, "Yemen: up to 85,000 young children dead from starvation" [Yemen: hasta 85 mil niños pequeños muertos de hambre], *The Guardian* (21 de noviembre de 2018), https://www.theguardian.com/world/2018/nov/21/yemen-young-children-dead-starvation-disease-save-the-children.

75. Joseph Hincks, "What you need to know about the crisis in Yemen" [Lo que hay que saber sobre la crisis en Yemen], *Time* (3 de noviembre de 2016), https://time.com/4552712/yemen-war-humanitarian-crisis-famine/.

76. Frederika Whitehead, Water scarcity in Yemen: the country's forgotten conflict, [La escasez de agua en Yemen: el conflicto olvidado del país] *The Guardian* (2 de abril de 2015, 5:18 a.m.), https://www.theguardian.com/global-development-professionals-network/2015/apr/02/water-scarcity-yemen-conflict; IRIN in Sana'a, "Time running out for solution to Yemen's water crisis" [Se acaba el tiempo para encontrar soluciones a la crisis del agua en Yemen], *The Guardian* (27 de agosto de 2012, 7:30 a.m.), https://www.theguardian.com/global-development/2012/aug/27/solution-yemen-water-crisis.

77. O'Brien Statement 2017, nota *supra* 71.

78. Alex De Waal, "The end of famine? Prospects for the elimination of mass starvation by political action," [¿El fin de la hambruna? Perspectivas para la eliminación del hambre masiva por medio de la acción política] *Political Geography* 62 (2018): 184, 185

79. *Id.* en 185.

alimentaria).[80] La gravedad de la inseguridad alimentaria consta de cinco fases: 1) mínima, 2) estresada, 3) crisis, 4) emergencia y 5) hambruna.[81] Varias regiones del Yemen se encuentran actualmente ya sea en la fase 3 de crisis o en la fase 4 de emergencia.[82] Las zonas con peor grado de inseguridad alimentaria son aquellos donde se libra el conflicto: Hudaydah, Sana'a, Ta' izz, Aden y las aldeas costeras del Mar Rojo.

Las muertes civiles en Yemen a causa del hambre y de enfermedades relacionadas con la misma, como el cólera, son ocasionadas por el hombre.[83] Dos categorías de eventos son las principalmente responsables de los decesos y las lesiones relacionados con el hambre: (1) los ataques militares en perjuicio de la producción agrícola y alimentaria que destruyen, niegan o inutilizan los bienes indispensables para la supervivencia y (2) los bloqueos aeroportuarios y marítimos que obstruyen el flujo de ayuda humanitaria.[84] Entre los grupos responsables de estas atrocidades se encuentran todas las principales partes del conflicto: los rebeldes hutíes apoyados por Irán, el gobierno y los militares yemeníes, así como la coalición militar liderada por Arabia Saudita (SLC, por sus siglas en inglés). La documentación de los ataques en perjuicio de los suministros de alimentos para los civiles demuestra que estos fueron blanco de ataques como parte de un método de guerra, lo que constituye una violación inequívoca del *jus in bello* y de la tradición de la Guerra Justa.[85] Existen informes que señalan que el príncipe heredero de Arabia Saudita, Mohammad bin Salman, autorizó la utilización del hambre como método de guerra para poder derrotar a los hutíes.[86]

---

80. Paul Howe y Stephen Deveraux, "Famine Intensity and Magnitude Scales: A proposal for an instrumental definition of famine," [Escalas de intensidad y magnitud de la hambruna: una propuesta para una definición instrumental de la hambruna] 28 (2004): 353–372; Famine Early Warning Systems Network, Integrated Phase Classification, https://fews.net/IPC.

81. Famine Early Warning Systems Network, "Integrated Phase Classification," [Red de sistemas de alerta temprana de la hambruna, "Clasificación de fase integrada"] https://fews.net/IPC.

82. Famine Early Warning Systems Network, "Yemen Food Security Outlook", de octubre de 2019 a mayo de 2020, https://fews.net/east-africa/yemen/food-security-outlook/october-2019.

83. *Véase, en general*, De Waal, nota *supra* 17.

84. Martha Mundy, "The Strategies of the Coalition in the Yemen War: Aerial Bombardment and Food War" [Las estrategias de la coalición en la guerra de Yemen: bombardeos aéreos y guerra alimentaria], *World Peace Foundation* 11 (2018), https://sites.tufts.edu/wpf/files/2018/10/Strategies-of-Coalition-in-Yemen-War-Final-20181005-1.pdf [en lo sucesivo Mundy].

85. *Id.* en 24.

86. Un diplomático de alto rango de la coalición liderada por Arabia Saudita declaró

En Yemen, uno de los principales factores para la generalización del hambre y las enfermedades derivadas de la misma, ha sido la destrucción deliberada y desproporcionada de los bienes indispensables para la supervivencia, incluyendo los ataques a infraestructuras clave como son las fuentes de electricidad, abastecimiento de agua, presas de riego, instalaciones de extensión agrícola e instalaciones sanitarias. El Consejo de Derechos Humanos de las Naciones Unidas informó que los ataques aéreos del SLC habían ocasionado daños considerables a bienes de carácter civil, lo que se traducía en numerosas muertes de civiles.[87] La destrucción de los bienes indispensables para la supervivencia en Ta'izz, Tihama y la costa del Mar Rojo son algunos de los incidentes más atroces de la guerra en Yemen que han provocado que los civiles padezcan hambre.

Puesto que era uno de los principales campos de batalla en el conflicto entre los rebeldes hutíes y el SLC, la gobernación de Ta'izz sufrió una de las mayores pérdidas humanas de la guerra. A principios del año 2014, los bienes de carácter civil fueron blanco de frecuentes ataques, los cuales provocaron la muerte y el desplazamiento de muchos civiles.[88] Diversos factores han hecho más grave la inseguridad alimentaria en Ta'izz, provocando con ello que los civiles padezcan hambre. Como resultado de la lucha constante, el acceso a los alimentos en los mercados ha disminuido significativamente y el precio de los alimentos ha subido de forma drástica, volviéndolos inaccesibles para muchas personas.[89] Además, los ataques aéreos de la SLC dirigidos a granjas, mercados, administraciones agrícolas y centros de transporte han empeorado aún más la escasez de alimentos.[90] En

---

extraoficialmente:"Una vez que los controlemos, los alimentaremos". *Id.* en 7; *Véase también* "Bin Salman threatens to target women and children in Yemen despite international criticism," [Bin Salman amenaza con atacar a mujeres y niños en Yemen a pesar de la crítica internacional] *Middle East Monitor* (27 de agosto de 2018, 10:39 a.m.), https://www. middleeastmonitor.com/20180827-bin-salman-threatens-to-target-women-and-children-in-yemen-despite-international-criticism/.

87. UN Office of the High Commissioner on Human Rights, *Yemen: United Nations Experts point to possible war crimes by parties to the conflict* [La oficina del Alto Comisionado de las Naciones Unidas para los Derechos Humanos, Yemen: Expertos de las Naciones Unidas señalan posibles crímenes de guerra por las partes en el conflicto] (28 de agosto de 2018), https://www.ohchr.org/EN/NewsEvents/Pages/DisplayNews.aspx?NewsID=23479.

88. World Peace Foundation, Accountability for Mass Starvation: World Peace Foundation [Fundación para la paz mundial, responsabilidad por el hambre: resumen de las políticas sobre el hambre en Yemen], 6–7 (2019), https://sites.tufts.edu/wpf/files/2019/06/Accountability-for-Starvation-Crimes-Yemen.pdf [en adelante, Resumen de las políticas de la Fundación para la paz mundial].

89. *Id.* en 6-7.

90. *Id.*

diciembre de 2017, la SLC lanzó ataques aéreos contra un mercado en el distrito de al-Ta 'iziyah, destruyéndolo por completo y dejando un saldo de cincuenta y cuatro civiles muertos y otros treinta y dos heridos.[91] En agosto de 2018, el 75% de la población civil de Ta'izz estaba clasificada dentro de los márgenes de la inseguridad alimentaria y al menos el 85% dependía de la ayuda humanitaria.[92]

Además de los ataques en Ta'izz, otras zonas del país, incluyendo algunas aldeas de pescadores han sido blanco de ataques. Entre marzo de 2015 y agosto de 2016 tuvieron lugar numerosos ataques aéreos contra objetivos agrícolas.[93] Los ataques a las tierras agrícolas son atroces en particular, puesto que solo el 5% de la tierra de Yemen es cultivable y, antes de la guerra, solo el 3% de la superficie total de Yemen era utilizada para la agricultura.[94] En Tihama, los ataques contra los bienes indispensables para la supervivencia no se perpetraron contra campos o granjas, sino contra sistemas de riego impulsados por bombeo de petróleo. Desde principios del año 2011 y como consecuencia de la guerra, la escasez del petróleo y el incremento de precios han hecho que a los agricultores les sea casi imposible regar sus tierras.[95]

Desde finales de la década de los setenta, el Banco Mundial ha invertido en estructuras de desviación de agua diseñadas profesionalmente, supervisadas por la Autoridad de Desarrollo de Tihama (TDA, por sus siglas en inglés), las cuales son utilizadas para fortalecer el suministro de agua a las granjas y a las tierras agrícolas de la región.[96] En dos ocasiones, en agosto de 2015 y nuevamente en septiembre, la SLC lanzó un total de quince ataques aéreos contra el complejo central de la TDA, a las afueras de Hudaydah y tres ataques aéreos más en contra de las estructuras de riego en Wadi Siham en octubre de ese mismo año.[97] El Proyecto de Datos de Yemen informa de dos ataques adicionales a la infraestructura de la TDA en 2016 y otros tres a principios de 2017.[98] Como consecuencia de estos ataques, la producción agrícola disminuyó un 24% entre los agricultores de Wadi Zabid y un 46%

---

91. *Id.*
92. *Id.*
93. Mundy, nota *supra* 84, en 11.
94. Organización de las Naciones Unidas para la Agricultura y la Alimentación, "Selected Indicators" [Indicadores selectos], http://www.fao.org/faostat/en/?#country/249.
95. Mundy, nota *supra* 84, en 13.
96. *Id.* en 14.
97. *Id.*
98. *Id.*

en Wadi Siham, debido principalmente, a la escasez de agua de riego.[99] En la región de Tihama, alguna vez considerada como el cuerno de la abundancia de Yemen, el cultivo de la tierra ha disminuido en un 51%, la productividad agrícola de los cultivos ha disminuido entre un 20 y un 61% por hectárea y las frutas, las verduras y el ganado han sido aniquilados por completo, lo que ha llevado al 43% de la población a padecer inseguridad alimentaria.[100]

La pesca artesanal ha sido durante mucho tiempo una fuente primaria de producción de alimentos en Yemen. La Autoridad General de Pesca en el Mar Rojo documentó daños a la actividad pesquera desde el comienzo de la guerra hasta diciembre de 2017, reportando 146 pescadores muertos y 220 barcos pesqueros destruidos durante ataques aéreos de la SLC en el año 2018.[101] En 2015, antes de la guerra, el sector pesquero de Yemen ocupaba el segundo lugar en términos de exportaciones y constituía el 2% del PIB yemení.[102]

Otra causa importante del hambre en Yemen es la obstrucción y manipulación ilegal de la ayuda humanitaria debido a los bloqueos. La evidencia de la obstaculización de los suministros y las operaciones humanitarias demuestran que los bloqueos han suspendido la entrega de asistencia humanitaria y que se han propiciado demoras injustificadas en el transporte de la misma hacia las áreas azotadas por la hambruna.

Hudaydah era la gobernación más pobre de Yemen antes de que estallara la guerra en el año 2015.[103] El 60% de la población de Yemen con algún grado de desnutrición residía en Hudaydah.[104] Existen tres puertos principales en la gobernación, dos de los cuales, Al-Hudaydah y Al-Saleef, reciben la mayoría de las importaciones alimentarias del país; el número total de las importaciones

---

99. The Water and Environment Center of San'a' University, *Food Production, Irrigation, Marketing, and Agricultural Coping Mechanisms, Tihama (Wadi Zabid and Wadi Siham), Briefing Note 2-Food Security* (FBLN, NICHE-Yem027), Flood-Based Livelihoods Network Foundation, http://spate-irrigation-org/wp-content/uploads/2018/02/Briefing-Note-2-%E2%80%93-Food-Security-pdf.

100. Flood-based Livelihoods Network Foundation, "Yemen's Burnt Granary," [El granero quemado de Yemen] http://spate-irrigation.org/yemens-burnt-granary/#more-6422.

101. Taqrir 'an al-qita ' al-samaki fi-'l-bahr al-ahmar ba' d alf yaum min al- 'udwan [Informe sobre el sector pesquero en el Mar Rojo luego de mil días de agresión] al-Hai' ah al-'Amman li' -Masa 'id al-Samakiya fi' l-Bahr al-Ahmar ,13–43 (enero de 2018).

102. Ammar Al-Fareh, "The Impact of the War in Yemen on Artisanal Fishing of the Red Sea" [El impacto de la guerra en Yemen sobre la pesca artesanal en el Mar Rojo, *LSE Middle East Centre Report* 7 (2018), http://eprints.lse.ac.uk/91022/1/Al-Fareh_The-impact-of-war_Author.pdf.

103. WPF Policy Brief, nota *supra* 88, en 7.

104. *Id.*

comerciales ha disminuido significativamente desde el año 2014.[105] Existen otros dos puertos en Yemen, en Adén y en Al-Mukalla, pero carecen de la infraestructura necesaria para la recepción de remesas de alimentos a granel.[106] En abril de 2015, la SLC emprendió un bloqueo contra los puertos del Mar Rojo con el fin de inspeccionar aquellos buques comerciales que pudieran transportar armas prohibidas para los huties.[107] El resultado del bloqueo, que duró dieciséis meses, fue limitar en forma efectiva el flujo de alimentos, combustible y medicinas destinadas para los civiles.[108] El 6 de noviembre de 2017, la SLC tomó represalias por un ataque de misiles tipo Houthi contra la ciudad de Riyadh, imponiendo a Yemen un bloqueo aéreo, marítimo y terrestre durante dieciséis días, durante el cual bloqueó todos los suministros de alimentos y combustibles que entraban al país,[109] lo que a su vez provocó que aumentara la inseguridad alimentaria y las muertes por hambre y desnutrición.

La guerra en Yemen constituye un caso de estudio muy distinto al del Plan del Hambre de los nazis. Mientras que los nazis utilizaron el hambre como arma de exterminio, la SLC utiliza los bloqueos y ataca los bastiones huties. Incluso si se demostrara que las tácticas de la SLC no propiciaron de manera intencional el hambre en la población civil o tenían como blanco específico los bienes indispensables para la supervivencia y su destrucción, lo que sería muy difícil de probar según las evidencias que se mencionaron anteriormente, estas tácticas son, a pesar de todo, actos *malum in se* puesto que tienen como resultado una profunda indiferencia ante el hambre de los civiles y suponen, además, la violación de los cuatro principios del DIH establecidos previamente. Así mismo, aunque los bloqueos y los ataques aéreos de la SLC en Yemen pudieran tener la intención de un buen efecto (por ejemplo, la derrota de los rebeldes huties y la restauración de la paz y la seguridad en la región), el mal efecto (el hambre) no se justifica bajo la tercera y cuarta condición del PDE, puesto que no es permisible usar un mal medio para lograr un buen fin, y el efecto de poner fin a la guerra, que de cualquier forma no ha funcionado, no es proporcional a la muerte por hambre de las personas civiles. Por estas razones, me pronuncio a favor de prohibiciones más estrictas en cuanto a los métodos legales de la guerra que de manera directa o indirecta propician el hambre.

---

105. *Id.*
106. *Id.* en 7-8.
107. *Id.*
108. *Id.* en 8.
109. *Id.*

Parte IV: Conclusión

En el presente ensayo se ha argumentado que, conforme al derecho internacional, el uso del hambre como método de guerra debe prohibirse totalmente por ser un acto *malum in se*. Si bien podría argumentarse que tanto el DIH como el ICL ya prohíben el hambre, sostengo que los instrumentos jurídicos actuales que la prohíben son inadecuados tanto porque no se cumplen, como porque los instrumentos actuales la permiten cuando se trata de una consecuencia indirecta de los métodos de guerra lícitos, como son los sitios y los bloqueos. Estos problemas ponen de relieve la necesidad de imponer mayores restricciones dentro del marco jurídico actual para garantizar que el hambre no sea nunca el resultado permisible de un objetivo militar, ya sea directa o indirectamente.

El problema del cumplimiento de la ley se debe en gran medida al hecho de que los ejemplos más recientes en los que se han cometido crímenes de hambre, como en Yemen y Siria, no están sujetos a la jurisdicción de la CPI. Sin una recomendación del Consejo de Seguridad de la ONU a la CPI, es muy poco probable que los autores de crímenes de hambre respondan[110] por ellos puesto que los sistemas legales de estos estados fallidos no pueden, o no quieren, procesar a los autores. Por ello, la mejor opción es la de preservar la evidencia de los crímenes de hambre para futuros enjuiciamientos y para que la comunidad internacional ejerza presión sobre los miembros del Consejo de Seguridad, pero en particular sobre los P3 (Estados Unidos, China y Rusia), para que aprueben una Resolución del Capítulo VII para la investigación de los crímenes de hambre en Yemen y en Siria, y recomienden el enjuiciamiento de los responsables.

Otra forma de poner fin a la utilización del hambre como arma de guerra es que los Estados hagan declaraciones condenatorias y exijan que la codificación o el desarrollo progresivo del derecho internacional imponga prohibiciones más estrictas sobre la utilización del hambre. Algunas estrategias para lograr este objetivo incluyen la tipificación del delito de provocación del hambre como una norma perentoria de *jus cogens* no derogable en virtud de los tratados y convenciones actuales,[111] y el cabildeo ante el Consejo de

---

110. Graham, nota *supra* 27.

111. La labor de la Comisión de Derecho Internacional sobre las normas perentorias del *jus cogens* del derecho internacional general no enumera la prohibición del hambre en su reciente informe, pero la prohibición de los crímenes de lesa humanidad y el genocidio están ciertamente estrechamente relacionados con el hambre. *Véase* Int'l Law Com., Normas perentorias del derecho internacional general (*jus cogens*), Texto preliminar de las conclusiones y el anexo adoptado provisionalmente por el Comité de Redacción en su primera lectura, (29 de mayo de 2019), A/CN.4/L.936.

Seguridad para que adopte una resolución conforme al Capítulo VII para que se ponga fin al hambre como arma de guerra y se le considere como *malum in se*. Estas medidas enviarían una señal clara de que, conforme al derecho internacional, ya no se tolerará el hambre.

Finalmente, los expertos en ética militar pueden influir para conseguir que la ley cambie persuadiendo a los funcionarios del Estado y a los líderes militares de que los métodos de guerra lícitos que propician el hambre, ya sea directa o indirectamente, no son necesarios para la consecución de los objetivos militares. Existen otros medios que pueden ayudar a la consecución de objetivos similares sin las insidiosas consecuencias del sufrimiento de las personas civiles a causa del hambre. Por lo tanto, un cambio de actitud entre los líderes militares y los funcionarios de Estado puede forjar una nueva costumbre de que el hambre es *malum in se*, facilitando la imposición de restricciones legales más serias con respecto a su utilización durante la guerra y poniendo fin a la impunidad de los autores de crímenes de hambre.

Malum in se
La famine comme crime de guerre dans le droit international

Laura K. Graham

La famine est employée comme une méthode de guerre depuis des temps immémoriaux. Or, depuis les cent-cinquante dernières années, en dépit des évolutions du droit des conflits armés (DCA) par des lois visant à l'interdiction de la famine intentionnelle en temps de guerre, la famine comme méthode de guerre perdure jusqu'à nos jours. Cela s'explique par le fait que les belligérants disposent de deux moyens légaux pouvant être des vecteurs de famine : (1) la guerre de siège et (2) les blocus ayant pour but de couper les vivres à l'ennemi. Dans ce travail, j'aborderai le fait que de telles tactiques ne sont jamais moralement justifiées et devraient donc être totalement prohibées, même dans les lieux où les belligérants emploient la famine intentionnelle sous le couvert du droit international humanitaire (DIH), car la faim est qualifiable de *malum in se* ; en l'occurrence, il s'agit d'un acte intrinsèquement immoral, qu'il soit ou non prohibé par le DIH. Il en est ainsi, car lorsque la faim est employée comme arme de guerre, c'est en violation des principes du *jus in bello*.

La première partie de ce travail fait l'examen du DIH d'un point de vue historique en évoquant l'expansion des interdictions, ainsi que des limites, s'appliquant à l'utilisation de la famine durant les conflits armés dans le droit pénal international (DPI), depuis le Code Lieber de 1863 jusqu'à l'amendement de 2019 du Statut de Rome qui interdit l'utilisation de la famine dans les conflits armés internes définissant cette dernière comme un crime de guerre. La deuxième partie défend l'argument que la famine intentionnelle est un exemple de *malum in se* (mal en soi), car elle contrevient à certains principes fondamentaux du *jus in bello* (droit dans la guerre) à savoir les notions de distinction, de proportionnalité, de nécessité et d'interdiction des maux superflus et des souffrances inutiles. Dans la troisième partie sont présentées deux études de cas—une, historique, la deuxième, récente—dans lesquelles la famine a été employée comme arme de guerre. Il s'agit de décrire tout d'abord le Plan de la faim nazi afin de souligner le caractère immoral qu'il y a à instrumentaliser la faim contre l'ennemi. Ensuite sera évoqué le cas récent de la guerre civile au Yémen où treize millions de personnes sont en proie au risque de famine ou à une mort possible suite à des maladies liées à la faim à cause des attaques de la coalition dirigée par l'Arabie saoudite dans les zones agricoles qui privent la population civile d'eau potable et de biens indispensables à sa survie. Ces études de cas sont censées démontrer que même sous couvert du droit, l'instrumentalisation de la faim comme arme de guerre est un exemple de *malum in se* et devrait être, en tant que telle, d'une part, totalement interdite et d'autre part, soumise à des sanctions sous couvert du droit international. Enfin, la conclusion de ce travail entend préconiser, en vertu du droit international, la mise en place d'interdictions plus strictes concernant le recours délibéré à la famine, tout en définissant des stratégies dans ce but.

Première partie. Évolutions historiques des limitations imposées à la famine comme méthode de guerre

Les lois de la guerre—*jus in bello* ou droit international humanitaire—régissent la conduite des parties en présence dans un conflit armé et les tactiques militaires licites dans une guerre juste.[1] Parmi les principes humanitaires fondamentaux du droit de la guerre au 19è et au 20è siècle figuraient les notions de nécessité militaire et de proportionnalité—soit l'idée que les parties impliquées dans un conflit armé ne devraient pouvoir soutenir une attaque que lorsque cette dernière est nécessaire dans le but de remplir un objectif militaire légitime, sans négliger la notion de proportionnalité afin d'atténuer les dommages infligés aux populations civiles.[2] Oppenheim,

---

1. On situe généralement les premiers développements du droit international humanitaire après qu'Henry Durant, témoin de la bataille de Solférino en 1859, a établi le mouvement de la Croix-Rouge. Le code Lieber est considéré comme le tout premier exemple de codification du droit de la guerre. Toutefois, le droit de la guerre et le droit international humanitaire, bien qu'invoqués de façon interchangeable, sont tout à fait distincts l'un de l'autre : la législation de Genève, dérivée des tous premiers Accords de Genève, représente des principes humanitaires de droit coutumier alors que le droit de la Haye provient des conférences de la paix de la Haye de 1899 et 1907, représentant des règles conventionnelles régissant la conduite de la guerre. Or, il est important de noter que la plupart des chercheurs en droit ne considèrent plus la législation de Genève et le droit de la Haye comme deux entités distinctes. Voir Amanda Alexander, "A Short History of International Humanitarian Law," *European J. of Int'l L.* 26 (2015): 109, 112–116
2. *See, e.g.*, Judith Gardam, *Necessity, Proportionality and the Use of Force by States* (Cambridge University Press 2004 e-book) 28–30 (expliquant que les notions de nécessité et de proportionnalité faisaient partie intégrante de la théorie de la guerre juste depuis le moyen-âge) ; General Order No. 100 (24 avril 1863) Code Lieber, Instructions de 1863 pour les armées en campagne des États-Unis d'Amérique, Arts. 14–16, https://avalon.law.yale.edu/19th_century/lieber.asp#sec1 [ci-après, Lieber Code].

dans un traité intitulé *International Law*, décrit les deux premiers principes du droit de la guerre—nécessité et humanité—comme une contradiction qu'il est indispensable de résoudre.[3] Le droit international humanitaire, sous forme de législation et de conventions, s'en est inspiré pour réconcilier les nécessités de la guerre avec la notion d'humanité.

Les interdictions portant sur l'utilisation *injustifiée* de la famine en tant que méthode de guerre remontent au code Lieber de 1863 qui reconnaît que la famine est licite quand il s'agit de précipiter la reddition de l'ennemi, mais que les victimes civiles doivent se voir accordées les notions de nécessité et de proportionnalité présentes dans le DIH ; la mort de civils doit donc être nécessaire et proportionnée à l'objectif militaire légitime à atteindre, tel mettre fin à une guerre.[4] Elaboré pour l'armée de l'Union durant la guerre de sécession, le code Lieber prescrit les notions suivantes :

> La guerre n'est pas menée que par les armes. Il est légal d'affamer le belligérant ennemi, armé ou non, afin de parvenir plus rapidement à la soumission de l'ennemi. Quand le commandant d'une place assiégée fait sortir les non-combattants pour diminuer le nombre des personnes vivant sur son stock de provisions, il est légal, bien que d'une extrême rigueur, de les repousser en vue de hâter la reddition.[5]

La nécessité militaire de faire usage de la famine intentionnelle pour précipiter une reddition est donc inhérente au code Lieber. On remarque que le recours au siège ou au blocus ne peut être licite qu'en cas de nécessité militaire légitime : en d'autres mots, il ne serait pas légitime d'utiliser la famine pour punir l'ennemi, pour exterminer sa population ou dans le but de pillages des territoires ennemis à des fins de saisie de nourriture et de matériel afin de prolonger une campagne militaire. Bien que le code Lieber ne décrive pas expressément la notion de proportionnalité, l'article 18 pourrait être interprété comme une disposition en vertu de la

---

3. *See, e.g.*, L. Oppenheim, *International Law: A Treatise*, edited by R. F. Roxburgh, 3rd ed. (1921), 84–85.

4. Lieber Code, *supra* note 3, at Arts. 17–18.

5. Lieber Code, *supra* note 3, at Arts. 17–18 (parties mises en italiques par mes soins). Les autorisations définies dans le code Lieber Code de repousser des combattants dans une zone assiégée afin de précipiter la défaite de l'ennemi entre en contradiction directe avec la convention moderne indiquant que, tant que possible, la population civile et les non-combattants doivent pouvoir quitter une zone de combat ou que des couloirs humanitaires doivent être ménagés pour eux. *Voir, par ex.*, Protocole additionnel aux Conventions de Genève du 12 août 1949 relatif à la protection des victimes de conflits armés internationaux (Protocole I), 8 juin 1977, Arts. 54, 70.

proportionnalité dans la mesure où l'objectif de la guerre de siège est de hâter la capitulation, limitant ainsi le nombre de victimes. Or, il manque au code Lieber le principe d'humanité, soit l'idée que la souffrance visant spécifiquement la population civile est illicite et injuste. En cela, il serait donc exagéré d'affirmer que le code Lieber est la première codification de la famine imposée aux civils, quoiqu'il pourrait être perçu comme un premier pas dans cette direction, étant donné les conditions de la nécessité militaire et de la proportionnalité suggérées dans les Articles 17–18.

Bien qu'aucune interdiction expresse de l'utilisation de la famine dans la population civile n'ait existé au 19è siècle, la Convention de la Haye de 1899 pourrait être interprétée comme une manière d'éviter la faim selon la clause de Martens qui interdit des méthodes de guerre à même de heurter la conscience publique.[6] Est prescrit par la clause de Martens, stipulée dans le préambule de la seconde conférence de la Haye en 1899 :

> En attendant qu'un code plus complet des lois de la guerre puisse être édicté, les Hautes Parties Contractantes jugent opportun de constater que, dans les cas non compris dans les dispositions réglementaires adoptées par Elles, *les populations et les belligérants restent sous la sauvegarde et sous l'empire des principes du droit des gens,* tels qu'ils résultent des usages établis entre nations civilisées, *des lois de l'humanité et des exigences de la conscience publique.*[7]

Le principe d'humanité est donc voulu comme un garde-fou censé empêcher les belligérants de se livrer à des guerres anti-humanitaires. Ce principe interdit les méthodes de guerre qui ne sont pas nécessaires à l'obtention d'un avantage militaire précis[8] ; en cela, il est intimement lié au principe interdisant les armes qui peuvent infliger des maux superflus.[9] Jean Pictet interpréta le principe d'humanité comme suit : « [L]es non-

---

6. Le principe d'humanité, parfois assimilé à la clause de Martens, protège les civils des violations du DIH n'étant pas expressément couvertes par les traités. Il fut introduit par Fyodor Fyodorovich Martens dans le préambule de la Conférence de la Haye de 1899. *Voir* ICRC, "Fundamental Principles of IHL," https://casebook.icrc.org/glossary/fundamental-principles-ihl.

7. Convention (II) with Respect to the Laws and Customs of War on Land and its annex: Regulations concerning the Laws and Customs of War on Land, The Hague, 29 July 1899, Preamble (italiques ajoutés par mes soins).

8. E. Kwakwa, *The International Law of Armed Conflict: Personal and Material Fields of Application* (Kluwer Academic, Dordrecht, 1992), 36.

9. Convention (II) with Respect to the Laws and Customs of War on Land and its annex: Regulations concerning the Laws and Customs of War on Land, The Hague, 29 July 1899, Preamble.

combattants doivent être épargnés autant que possible » [10]. Une interprétation plus large consiste à penser que même si un traité ou une convention
n'interdit pas expressément un acte donné ou une conduite spécifique de
la part des belligérants, cela n'implique pas que l'acte ou la conduite en
question soit autorisé *ipso facto*. Au contraire, acte ou conduite sont assujet-
tis aux principes du droit coutumier international.[11] Dans le cadre de la
famine, on peut faire valoir la notion suivante : bien qu'aucun traité ou
convention n'ait expressément interdit la famine intentionnelle des civils
durant la deuxième guerre mondiale, le principe d'humanité de Martens
suggère que l'utilisation de la famine comme méthode de guerre n'était
pas destinée à remplir un quelconque objectif militaire légitime ni n'était
proportionnée, et de ce fait, était donc illégale selon la coutume de l'époque.

En outre, la Convention de la Haye de 1907 ne mentionne pas expressément la famine comme une méthode de guerre, mais prescrit que la guerre
de siège, qui a pour effet d'affamer les civils et les combattants, est licite.[12] La
Convention de la Haye de 1907 réitère le principe d'humanité défini par la
clause de Martens ainsi que le principe de nécessité.[13] Aussi cette convention
pourrait-elle être interprétée comme l'interdiction d'une tactique militaire
telle que le Plan de la faim nazi qui utilisait la famine intentionnelle pour
éliminer la population civile plutôt que pour mettre fin à la guerre.

C'est d'ailleurs dans ce but que le Tribunal militaire international de
Nuremberg (TMI Nuremberg) a déclaré que le droit de la guerre défini

---

10. Jean Pictet, *Development and Principles of International Humanitarian Law*, Martinus
Nijhoff and Henry Dunant Institute (Dordrecht/Geneva, 1985), 62.
11. Rupert Ticehurst, "The Martens Clause and the Laws of Armed Conflict," *International
Review of the Red Cross* 317 (Apr. 30, 1997), https://casebook.icrc.org/glossary/
fundamental-principles-ihl ; *But see*, S. S. Lotus (Fr. v. Turk.), Judgment, 1927 P.C.I.J. Series
A 16 No. 10 (Sept. 7), at 19 (Dans ses remarques incidentes, la cour décrit ce qui est connu
comme the second Lotus Principle, soit l'arrêt Lotus, lequel suggère que tout ce qui n'est
pas expressément interdit par le droit international est autorisé : « Mais il ne s'ensuit pas que
le droit international défend à un État d'exercer, dans son propre territoire, sa juridiction
dans toute affaire où il s'agit de faits qui se sont passés à l'étranger et où il ne peut s'appuyer
sur une règle permissive du droit international. Pareille thèse ne saurait être soutenue que si
le droit international défendait, d'une manière générale, aux États d'atteindre par leurs lois
et de soumettre à la juridiction de leurs tribunaux des personnes, des biens et des actes hors
du territoire […] ».
12. L'Article 27 de la Convention (IV) de la Haye pose des interdictions à l'encontre des
belligérants concernant l'attaque des malades et des blessés durant un siège, mais cette
interdiction ne s'adresse pas spécifiquement aux civils, et l'Article 28 interdit de se livrer
au pillage d'une ville ou localité même prise d'assaut. *Voir* Convention (IV) respecting the
Laws and Customs of War on Land and its annex: Regulations concerning the Laws and
Customs of War on Land. The Hague, 18 October 1907, Arts. 27–28 [hereinafter, Hague
Convention IV].
13. *Id.* at Preamble.

par la Convention de la Haye de 1907 faisait partie du droit coutumier international en 1939 :

> « Les Règles la guerre terrestre contenues dans la Convention [de la Haye de 1907] réalisaient certes un progrès du Droit international (...) En 1939, ces règles, contenues dans la Convention, furent admises par tous les États civilisés et regardées par eux comme l'expression codifiée des lois et coutumes de la guerre... » [14]

Cependant, en dépit du fait que la Convention de la Haye de 1907 eut interdit aux belligérants de causer des souffrances inutiles et d'occasionner la destruction des propriétés ennemies,[15] le TMI Nuremberg mit en accusation non pas les Nazis pour crime de famine intentionnelle lié au Plan de la faim, mais le feld-maréchal Wilhelm von Leeb pour le siège de Leningrad dans le procès dit « des grands criminels de guerre ». Ce procès, comme son nom l'indique, consistait en des poursuites judiciaires contre douze officiers du Haut-Commandement Nazi pour crimes de guerre et crimes contre la paix durant la deuxième guerre mondiale. Celui de von Leeb s'appliquait à son rôle dans l'invasion de l'Union Soviétique pendant l'opération Barbarossa. C'est ainsi que le verdict rendu par le TMI Nuremberg indiquait qu'en dépit du fait que la famine occasionnée par le siège fût flagrante, elle était néanmoins légale :

> Un commandant belligérant peut légalement assiéger une région contrôlée par l'ennemi et s'efforcer, par un processus d'isolement, de provoquer sa reddition. Le bien-fondé qu'il y a à tenter de l'y réduire par la famine n'est pas remis en question. On dit que si le commandant d'une place assiégée expulse les non-combattants afin de diminuer le nombre des personnes vivant sur son stock de provisions, *il est légal, bien que d'une extrême rigueur, de les repousser en vue de hâter la reddition.* ...C'est pourquoi l'isolation de toute source de subsistance venant de l'extérieur est considérée comme légitime.... *Nous pourrions souhaiter que la loi soit différente, mais il est de notre devoir de l'appliquer telle que nous la trouvons.* Par conséquent, nous ne retenons aucune responsabilité pénale à l'égard de cette accusation.[16]

---

14. International Military Tribunal at Nuremberg, reprinted in *AJIL* 41, 248–249 (1947).

15. Hague Convention IV, *supra* note 12, at Art. 23.

16. Trials of War Criminals before the Nuernberg Military Tribunals Under Control Council Law No. 10, Nuernberg, October 1946–April 1949, Vol. XI, 563 (U.S. Government Printing Office, Washington, D.C., 1950) (italiques ajoutés par mes soins).

En effet, la pratique des États suggère que les parties en présence lors de la deuxième guerre mondiale, à l'exception de l'Union Soviétique, croyaient unanimement que la famine organisée dans le but de forcer l'ennemi à la capitulation constituait une méthode de guerre légitime et légale. Par exemple, les États-Unis et le Royaume-Uni firent usage de blocus alimentaires en Allemagne, dans les territoires occupés par l'Allemagne et au Japon ; les États-Unis allèrent jusqu'à nommer leur blocus portuaire au Japon « Opération Famine ».[17] Ainsi, la famine causée par sièges et blocus n'étaient pas interdites *ipso facto* selon le droit international pendant la seconde guerre mondiale. Toutefois, le fait que la famine comme arme de guerre n'était pas strictement prohibée durant cette période n'établit pas que l'utilisation de la famine fût conforme aux principes de nécessité militaire, de proportionnalité, de distinction ou d'humanité.

Des exactions commises durant la seconde guerre mondiale il est sorti deux évolutions majeures dans le droit international : la Convention sur le génocide de 1948 et la Convention de Genève pour la protection des populations civiles de 1949 qui interdisent expressément la famine intentionnelle des civils comme arme de guerre.[18] La Convention sur le génocide interdit la « Soumission intentionnelle du groupe à des conditions d'existence devant entraîner sa destruction physique totale ou partielle. »[19] Il est indéniable que la famine intentionnelle entre dans ce critère. Plus récemment le Protocole additionnel de la Convention de Genève de 1977 donne des explications détaillées au sujet des autorisations et des interdictions portant sur les sièges, les blocus, les atteintes aux biens indispensables à la survie de population et l'aide humanitaire.[20] De plus, le Statut de Rome de 1998[21] et ses amendements de 2019 incriminent la famine comme arme de guerre en cas de conflits internationaux et non internationaux.[22] En particulier l'Article 54 du

---

17. Alex De Waal, *Mass Starvation: The History and Future of Famine* (2018), 127–28.

18. Convention on the Prevention and Punishment of the Crime of Genocide, 9 December 1948, 78 U.N.T.S. 277, Art. II(c); Geneva Convention relative to the protection of civilian persons in time of war, Geneva 8 December 1949.

19. *Id.*

20. Protocol Additional to the Geneva Conventions of 12 August 1949 and Relating to the Protection of Victims of International Armed Conflicts (Protocol I), June 8, 1977, 1125 U.N.T.S. 3, at Art. 54(1) [hereinafter, Protocol I]; Protocol Additional to the Geneva Conventions of 12 August 1949 and relating to the Protection of Victims of Non-International Armed Conflict, June 8, 1977, 1125 U.N.T.S. 609, at Arts. 14, 69–70 [hereinafter, Protocol II].

21. Rome Statute of the International Criminal Court, Art. 8(2)(b)(xxv), 17 July 1998, UN Doc. A/CONF. 183/9, 2187 U.N.T.S. 9 [hereinafter, Rome Statute].

22. International Criminal Court Assembly of State Parties, Report of the Working Group

Protocole additionnel (I) et l'Article 14 du Protocole additionnel (II) interdisent les atteintes portées aux biens indispensables à la survie de la population
et la famine intentionnelle de la population civile alors que l'Article 70 du
Protocole additionnel (I) exige l'accès sans entrave à l'aide humanitaire.[23]
Quoique la famine des populations civiles soit strictement prohibée selon
l'Article 54, sièges et blocus constituent des exceptions à cette interdiction tant que l'attaque se conforme aux principes de nécessité militaire, de
distinction et de proportionnalité et ne prive pas la population civile de
nourriture et d'eau ou encore ne force pas les civils à quitter leur pays à cause
d'un manque de nourriture et d'eau.[24] Enfin, le Statut de Rome de la Cour
pénale internationale (CPI) donne à la famine le statut de crime de guerre
lorsque l'instigateur entend réduire la population civile à la famine comme
une méthode de guerre, priver les civils des biens indispensables à leur survie
ou empêcher délibérément les approvisionnements de secours.[25]

Bien que le droit ait évolué vers de plus importantes restrictions des
méthodes de guerre engendrant la famine, le droit international humanitaire
(DIH), le droit pénal international (DPI) et le droit international coutumier
ne sont pas en mesure de garantir une interdiction absolue de l'utilisation de
la famine en tant qu'arme de guerre. De ce fait, toute avancée du droit dans
ce sens devra résulter d'évolutions progressives. Comme il sera démontré
dans la suite de ce travail, la famine intentionnelle devrait être totalement
bannie sous le couvert du droit international, car elle est un exemple de
malum in se. Sera également invoquée la doctrine du double effet pour
soutenir les arguments qui suivront. En tant qu'exercice philosophique,
cette doctrine justifie le caractère licite d'actions néfastes, telle la famine
intentionnelle imposée à la population civile, en tant qu'effet secondaire de
bonnes intentions, comme celle de mettre fin à une guerre prolongée. À
savoir que quatre conditions doivent être remplies pour qu'une action soit
moralement licite sous le couvert de la doctrine du double effet :

1. L'action elle-même doit être bonne ou moralement neutre

---

on Amendments, Eighteenth session, 2–7 December 2019, 7–9, ICC-ASP/18/32 (Dec. 3,
2019), https://asp.icc-cpi.int/iccdocs/asp_docs/ASP18/ICC-ASP-18-32-ENG.pdf.
23. Protocol I, *supra* note 20, at arts. 54(1) & 70; Protocol II, *supra* note 20, at art. 14.
24. *Id.* at Additional Protocol I, art. 54(3).
25. Rome Statute, *supra* note 21, at art. 8(2)(b)(xxv)("Intentionally using starvation as a
method of warfare by depriving civilians of objects indispensable to their survival, including
willfully impeding relief supplies as provided for under the Geneva Conventions.");
See also Elements of Crimes, International Criminal Court (2001), at art. 8(2)(b)(xxv),
https://www.icc-cpi.int/nr/rdonlyres/336923d8-a6ad-40ec-ad7b-45bf9de73d56/0/
elementsofcrimeseng.pdf.

2. Le bon effet doit résulter de l'acte et non du mauvais effet.

3. Le mauvais effet ne doit pas être directement voulu, mais doit être prévu et toléré

4. Le bon effet doit être plus fort que le mauvais effet ou bien les deux doivent être égaux (au sens où ce serait un mal plus grand de l'éviter sans produire le bon effet).[26]

Une campagne de famine intentionnelle échappe clairement à la première condition énoncée, car la famine n'est jamais ni bonne ni moralement indifférente. Même la tactique du blocus pourrait être perçue comme moralement indifférente, si l'effet désiré du blocus en question était d'occasionner la famine pour mettre fin à la guerre, si ce n'est que dans ce cas, le blocus n'obéit pas à la troisième condition, car un mauvais effet (ici, la famine) ne doit jamais être utilisé dans le but d'obtenir un bon effet (à savoir empêcher que des armes ne tombent aux mains des ennemis).

Deuxième partie : Utilisation de la famine et malum in se

L'utilisation de la famine comme une méthode de guerre ressort du *malum in se* en ce qu'elle contrevient aux principes de distinction, de proportionnalité, de nécessité et de maux superflus inscrits dans le *jus in bello*.

La famine comme arme de guerre contrevient au principe de distinction du *jus in bello*

La famine intentionnelle est une arme qui ne fait fondamentalement aucune distinction entre les gens. Or, le DIH stipule que les civils puissent être distingués des combattants lors d'attaques militaires. Lorsque la famine est employée de manière licite, soit par siège soit par blocus, cette distinction devient caduque. C'est pourquoi les protocoles additionnels requièrent des combattants (1) qu'ils permettent la distribution de l'aide humanitaire aux civils durant les sièges et les blocus et/ou (2) qu'ils permettent aux civils de quitter les villes assiégées. De même, une attaque légale ciblant un territoire ennemi peut occasionner une famine quand elle détruit les biens indispensables à la survie de la population civile. Du fait qu'il s'agisse d'attaques aveugles et étant donné que les ressources en eau et les zones agricoles sont utilisées par les civils et par les combattants, la destruction des biens indispensables à la survie pour forcer la reddition de l'ennemi s'inscrit également dans le *malum in se*.

---

26. Stephen Coleman, *Military Ethics: An Introduction with Case Studies* (Oxford University Press 2012), 22.

D'aucuns soutiendront qu'utiliser légalement la famine, telle qu'elle peut être causée par sièges, blocus ou attaques portées sur les biens indispensables à la survie afin de cibler les combattants, ne ressort pas du *malum in se* tant que la souffrance des civils est contenue. Dans ce cas, le problème n'est pas tant que les sièges, les blocus ou les attaques par opérations militaires portées sur les biens indispensables à la survie puissent toucher les civils des combattants sans distinction, mais plutôt que les combattants eux-mêmes fassent le choix délibéré de ne pas opérer de distinction entre les civils et les combattants ennemis. Ces mauvais joueurs, qui contreviennent ainsi au DCA, devraient être sanctionnés selon les dispositions des Conventions de Genève ou du Statut de Rome.

La réalité de la situation est que même les combattants dits « bien intentionnés » participant à des sièges, des blocus et des attaques ne sont pas en mesure d'offrir la garantie absolue que de telles tactiques ne causeront pas de souffrance aux civils. En cela, les méthodes de guerre engendrant la famine vont à l'encontre de la quatrième condition de la doctrine du double effet, à savoir que le soi-disant « bon » effet de la capitulation forcée de l'ennemi n'est pas suffisamment souhaitable pour compenser le mauvais effet causant la souffrance infligée à la population civile par la famine généralisée. De plus, dans de nombreux cas, si ce n'est dans la majorité, l'aide humanitaire ne parvient pas à rejoindre les civils parce qu'elle est dérobée par les belligérants ou détruite pendant le transport. En outre, les civils ne sont pas toujours en mesure de quitter les villes assiégées. Les personnes âgées ou en situation de handicap et les jeunes enfants, à qui sont dus, d'un point de vue légal et éthique, des devoirs spécifiques de soins adaptés, sont limitées dans leurs déplacements et n'ont souvent pas d'endroit où se réfugier. Ainsi, même avec les meilleures intentions, les civils souffrent d'irréparables dommages lorsque sièges, blocus ou attaques portés sur les biens indispensables à la survie des populations civiles sont employés en tant qu'armes de guerre. Cet état de fait a été mis en évidence par les nombreux cas de famine recensés durant des conflits armés lors des cent dernières années, spécialement dans les conflits récents au Soudan, en Syrie et au Yémen où des centaines de milliers de civils sont morts de faim et de maladies causées par la faim à cause de la guerre.[27]

---

27. *See* Jennifer Trahan, *Existing Legal Limits to Security Council Veto Power in the Face of Atrocity Crimes*, 278–79 (Cambridge University Press 2020); *See also*, Laura Graham, "Pathways to Accountability for Starvation Crimes in Yemen," *Case Western J. of Intl. L.* 53 (2020).

La famine comme arme de guerre contrevient au principe de proportionnalité du *jus in bello*

La famine occasionne souvent des pertes et dommages excessifs. Le principe de proportionnalité du *jus in bello* interdit aux combattants de lancer une attaque ou d'employer tout autre moyen de guerre pouvant entraîner des pertes civiles excessives. Que certains sièges, blocus ou attaques sur les biens indispensables à la survie de la population civile soient légaux ou non, ils causent souvent d'énormes pertes parmi les civils. Le Plan de la faim Nazi entraîna ainsi la mort de plus de quatre millions de personnes,[28] tout comme la guerre civile en cours au Yémen expose actuellement treize millions de personnes à l'insécurité alimentaire pouvant entraîner morts par malnutrition sévère et maladies liées à la famine.[29] Dans le cadre du Plan de la faim, selon lequel les Nazis entendaient nourrir l'armée allemande en pillant les ressources alimentaires de l'Union Soviétique, les 4,7 millions de victimes recensées ne relèvent pas de la proportionnalité d'un objectif militaire légitime ; de même, on ne peut trouver de justification à cette situation selon la seconde condition de la doctrine du double effet stipulant que le bon effet doit résulter de l'acte et non du mauvais effet. Les Nazis ne visaient en aucun cas un bon effet. En mettant à contribution une étude de cas donnée, la troisième partie de ce travail s'attachera à démontrer que si l'objectif du Plan de la faim (nourrir l'armée allemande) pouvait être perçu comme légitime, d'autres conditions ayant été préalablement remplies, le but premier de ce plan était visiblement d'exterminer les Soviétiques. Il s'agit là de l'extermination d'un groupe national ou ethnique, soit d'un génocide, qui est toujours *malum in se*. Quant aux treize millions de personnes exposées au risque de famine au Yémen à cause de blocus et d'attaques portées sur les biens indispensables à la survie des populations civiles, mêmes si ces tactiques relèvent d'un objectif militaire légitime, le nombre de civils exposés au risque de possibles maladies et à la mort (soient 45% de la population),[30] est excessif et donc, disproportionné par rapport audit objectif.

Un contre-argument vient à l'encontre de l'idée que la famine en tant que méthode de guerre est disproportionnée, c'est-à-dire que la famine pourrait sauver la vie de gens innocents lorsqu'elle est utilisée pour hâter

---

28. De Waal, *supra* note 17, at 104.
29. BBC News, "Yemen could be 'worst famine in 100 years,'" (Oct. 15, 2018), https://www.bbc.com/news/av/world-middle-east-45857729.
30. The World Bank, "Total Population Yemen," https://data.worldbank.org/indicator/SP.POP.TOTL?locations=YE.

la reddition de l'ennemi. Dans la même veine, de nombreux historiens de guerre sont d'avis que l'utilisation de la famine contre les Allemands durant la première et la seconde guerre mondiale a précipité leur capitulation, épargnant ainsi de très nombreuses vies humaines.[31] D'aucuns soutiendront que si de semblables tactiques hâtent la capitulation de l'ennemi par comparaison à une campagne militaire soutenue, il faut alors considérer que les pertes civiles liées aux sièges, aux blocus et à la destruction de biens indispensables à la survie sont proportionnées à celles, plus importantes, qui auraient été occasionnées par un conflit prolongé.

Toutefois, pour mieux évaluer la perte de vies humaines liée à la famine durant les deux conflits mondiaux, il est nécessaire d'élargir la période considérée. En effet, les pertes humaines parmi les civils ne sont pas encourues dans les jours ou les mois qui suivent un siège ou un blocus, mais doivent être calculées sur la base des mois et, parfois, des années d'insécurité alimentaire et de maladies causées par le siège ou le blocus après la fin de la guerre. Dans l'Allemagne de 1916–17, « L'hiver des navets » qui fut causé en partie par des embargos américains, causa la mort d'au moins 750.000 Allemands touchés par la malnutrition, entraînant également une nette chute du taux de natalité durant cette période.[32] À savoir que nombre de ces morts eurent lieu six mois *après* l'armistice.[33] Pendant la seconde guerre mondiale, au moins vingt millions de personnes périrent de la faim, de malnutrition et de maladies y étant liées.[34] Inclus dans ce chiffre figurent un million de personnes décédées durant le siège de Leningrad.[35] Dans ce contexte, il est évident que les pertes civiles sont plus importantes qu'elles n'auraient dû l'être d'après le principe de proportionnalité.

La famine comme arme de guerre contrevient au principe de nécessité du *jus in bello*

La famine intentionnelle n'est jamais nécessaire en temps de guerre. Inscrit dans le *jus in bello*, le principe de nécessité permet l'utilisation d'autres mesures vraiment nécessaires à l'accomplissement d'un objectif militaire légitime. Par exemple, empêcher que des armes et des ressources diverses puissent tomber entre les mains de l'ennemi constitue un objectif militaire

---

31. *See generally,* Lizzie Collingham, *The Taste of War: World War II and the Battle for Food* (2012).
32. *Id.* at 25.
33. De Waal, *supra* note 17, at 74.
34. Collingham, *supra* note 31, at 2.
35. *Id.* at 5.

légitime pouvant être atteint par blocus. Toutefois, quand les blocus peuvent aussi entraver l'acheminement de l'aide humanitaire destinée aux populations civiles ou l'accès à des réserves de nourriture et d'eau, ces méthodes de guerre sont moralement répréhensibles parce qu'elles causent une souffrance et des maux inutiles aux civils. De plus, comme l'objectif militaire légitime ne peut pas être atteint de manière éthique par des moyens moralement corrompus, la famine, soit-elle une conséquence directe ou indirecte d'une méthode de guerre légale, ne peut satisfaire au principe de nécessité.

Les opposants à l'interdiction totale des sièges, blocus et autres méthodes de guerre légales utilisant la tactique de la famine sont persuadés que de telles interdictions ôteraient aux militaires une arme essentielle pourtant nécessaire dans quelques rares cas. Par exemple, quand la défaite militaire semble inévitable, si ce n'est par le recours au siège ou au blocus appliqué à un bastion tenu par les troupes ennemies afin d'empêcher leur approvisionnement en munitions, de tels moyens de guerre pourraient être perçus comme une nécessité. Contrairement au viol ou au génocide, qui sont *mala in se* en ce qu'ils ne sont jamais légitimes,[36] ces opposants, dans le cas du siège ou du blocus, pourraient avancer dans certains rares cas tels que "l'urgence suprême"[37] que la famine est non seulement un moindre mal, mais est également justifiée afin d'éviter une tragédie plus importante ou la défaite. De plus, quand le bien-fondé d'un objectif militaire l'emporte de manière significative sur les victimes civiles de la famine, l'utilisation de la famine est alors légitimée par le principe de nécessité.

Bien qu'il existe de rares cas d'urgence suprême justifiant des mesures extrêmes afin d'éviter l'extermination d'êtres humains, il y aura toujours, en réalité, des alternatives aux sièges, aux blocus et aux attaques sur les biens indispensables à la survie des populations civiles. D'après la seconde condition de la doctrine du double effet, l'action n'est pas justifiée si le bon effet (la victoire militaire) pouvait être atteint sans le mauvais effet (la famine). De plus, dans l'analyse de Orend, le concept de l'urgence suprême, tel qu'il est défini par Walzer, nuit à la tradition de la guerre juste en faisant fi des justifications morales énoncées dans les exigences du *jus in bello*.[38] Selon cette logique, la famine en tant que méthode de guerre ne pourrait en aucune manière trouver une légitimité, même en cas d'urgence suprême, car laisser

---

36. *See* Morten Dige, *Explaining the Principle of Mala in Se, J. Mil. Ethics* 11(2012), 318–332, 319.

37. Michael Walzer, *Just and Unjust Wars*, 252 (1977).

38. Brian Orend, *The Morality of War*, 147–148 (2006); *See also*, Martin Cook, "Michael Walzer's Concept of 'Supreme Emergency,'" *J. Mil. Ethics* 6 (2007):138–151, 143.

se dérouler un tel acte de malfaisance constituerait une sape en bonne et due forme des fondements moraux des principes du *jus in bello*. Ainsi, bien que la famine constitue une méthode efficace pour amener l'ennemi à la capitulation, il ne s'agit pas d'une nécessité militaire avérée, même dans les circonstances les plus effroyables. Même si la famine comme méthode de guerre pouvait effectivement représenter une nécessité avérée à cause d'une menace existentielle, la souffrance causée par une telle méthode est intrinsèquement malfaisante et doit absolument être prohibée. Par conséquent, l'argument défendant la nécessité de l'urgence suprême n'est pas convaincant, car réduire des innocents à la famine est un acte délétère en substance qui ne peut jamais être justifié sous couvert des exigences du *jus in bello*.[39]

La famine intentionnelle comme arme de guerre contrevient au principe de maux superflus du *jus in bello*

La famine cause des souffrances inutiles et des maux superflus aux civils et aux combattants. Au même titre que les mines, les armes à sous-munitions, les armes biologiques ainsi que d'autres armes illégales car ayant des effets pernicieux, la famine intentionnelle est un outil de guerre insidieux. La mort causée par la famine est lente et atroce. Il faut environ deux mois à un humain pour mourir de faim.[40] D'après Lizzie Collingham, qui fait des recherches sur l'alimentation en temps de guerre :

> Les victimes de famine meurent de dystrophie nutritionnelle, un processus selon lequel l'organisme ayant utilisé toutes ses réserves de graisse, les muscles fondent pour fournir les besoins énergétiques du corps. L'intestin grêle s'atrophie et les victimes ont de plus en plus de mal à métaboliser les nutriments contenus dans les faibles quantités de nourritures qu'ils parviennent à obtenir. Alors, l'organisme active un mécanisme de défense réduisant l'activité des organes vitaux comme le cœur et les reins et la victime souffre ainsi non seulement de faiblesse musculaire accrue mais également d'une fatigue plus générale et envahissante… La quantité d'eau présente dans l'organisme diminuant plus lentement que la fonte des muscles et des tissus, le corps devient flaccide. Certaines victimes de famine présentent des œdèmes par carences alimentaires qui font enfler leur corps par rétention d'eau. Les gonflements se situent d'abord au niveau de l'abdomen et des membres inférieurs pour ensuite se propager au reste du corps.

---

39. *See, e.g.,* Dige, *supra* note 36, at 319.
40. De Waal, *supra* note 17, at 21.

L'épiderme est alors étiré, luisant et très fragilisé. La pression artérielle baisse dangereusement ; la victime souffre de kératite (rougeurs et douleurs de la cornée), de douleurs aux gencives, de douleurs dans les membres inférieurs, de douleurs névralgiques, de tremblements et d'ataxie (soit une perte de contrôle de ses membres). Ces symptômes s'accompagnent d'envies irrésistibles de carbohydrates et de sel, ainsi que de diarrhées incontrôlables. Dans le laps de temps précédant la mort imminente, la victime ressent par intermittences une très forte dépression et des moments d'irritation intense pour tomber par la suite dans une torpeur profonde. Finalement, l'organisme n'a plus d'autre alternative que de se maintenir en vie en puisant des protéines dans ses organes vitaux…Le cœur, en particulier, s'atrophie…La défaillance des organes est la cause ultime de la mort. [41]

Aucun gain militaire ne peut justifier l'utilisation de cette arme pernicieuse. D'aucuns soutiendront que l'humanité utilise la famine intentionnelle comme arme de guerre depuis des millénaires et que si celle-ci était si terrible, d'une part, elle ne serait plus tolérée en temps de guerre et, d'autre part, les auteurs de crimes de guerre se verraient traduits en justice. Au demeurant, personne n'a jamais été jugé pour crime de famine intentionnelle. L'absence d'interdictions formelles et de poursuites pourraient d'ailleurs constituer la preuve que la communauté internationale trouve cette tactique acceptable, ou du moins plus facilement acceptable que les mines, les armes à sous-munitions et les armes biologiques. En outre, on peut soutenir l'argument qui consiste à penser que la mort de combattants occasionnée par la famine n'est pas pire que celles qui sont causées par des bombardements ou d'autres moyens légaux de faire la guerre. En effet, comme l'objectif des sièges et des blocus n'est pas spécifiquement d'affamer l'ennemi jusqu'à ce que mort s'ensuive, mais plutôt, de l'affamer jusqu'à la soumission et la reddition, les effets pernicieux de la famine dans les dernières étapes de la défaillance des organes est une occurrence improbable puisque l'ennemi se rend généralement bien avant d'en arriver à ce stade.

Toutefois il s'agit d'un argument fallacieux, vu que l'absence de poursuites à l'encontre des auteurs des crimes de famine intentionnelle est un problème de volonté politique et une impasse politique au Conseil de sécurité des Nations Unies, et non le reflet d'un défaut de perception des horreurs de la famine parmi ses membres. En effet, le fait que la communauté internationale

---

41. Collingham, *supra* note 31, at 5–6.

n'ait pas pris de mesures pour mettre fin aux blocus et aux attaques sur les biens indispensables à la survie des populations civiles au Yémen n'indique en rien qu'il n'y a pas eu d'effort concerté en ce sens. En effet, le Conseil de sécurité de l'ONU a voté la Résolution 2417 dans un effort de condamner la famine provoquée par la guerre au Yémen. De même, l'Amendement du Statut de Rome de 2019 élargit la notion de crime de guerre lié à la famine intentionnelle désormais applicable aux conflits armés non-internationaux.[42] L'absence de poursuites judiciaires pour crimes de famine intentionnelle est le simple reflet de la géopolitique de l'ordre mondial actuel. Alors qu'il pourrait n'y avoir aucune tentative infaillible de sauver le Yémen, à plus long terme la justice penche vers des restrictions de plus en plus sévères et éventuellement vers des interdictions formelles quant au recours à la famine comme méthode de guerre. Il faut ajouter qu'aucun exemple historique ne corrobore l'idée que l'ennemi capitule nécessairement avant que les effets pernicieux de la famine intentionnelle ne se mettent en place. En effet, durant les sièges ou les blocus, les ennemis combattants ont tendance à faire des réserves de rations d'eau et de nourriture pour leurs troupes, ce qui ne fait qu'augmenter la détresse des civils dans les zones de guerre. En tout état de cause, ce sont les civils qui souffrent le plus au cours de sièges et de blocus à cause des quantités limitées de nourriture et d'eau, du manque d'accès à l'eau potable et parce que les civils soumis à la famine sont plus souvent de jeunes enfants, des personnes âgées, des infirmes et des femmes enceintes, soient des populations qui sont moins à même de tolérer le manque de nourriture durant des périodes pro-longées. Quel que soit le nombre de personnes mourant de faim, le principe de maux superflus interdit la souffrance inutile ; de même, la mort par famine intentionnelle est une façon de mourir marquée d'une intolérable cruauté.

Troisième partie : Études de cas : Plan de la faim nazi et guerre civile au Yémen

Le Plan de la faim

Il est un fait établi que la capitulation des Allemands à l'issue de la Pre-mière Guerre mondiale est due à la faim, le manque d'approvisionnement

---

42. S.C. Res. 2417, ¶¶ 5–7 (May 24, 2018); International Criminal Court Assembly of State Parties, Report of the Working Group on Amendments, Eighteenth session, 2–7 December 2019, 7–9, ICC-ASP/18/32 (Dec. 3, 2019), https://asp.icc-cpi.int/iccdocs/asp_docs/ASP18/ICC-ASP-18-32-ENG.pdf. Assemblée des États Parties de la Cour Pénale Internationale, XVIIIè session, Rapport du Groupe de travail sur les amendements, 2 au 7 décembre 2019.

alimentaire ayant entravé l'accomplissement de leurs objectifs militaires.[43] Environ 750.000 Allemands sont morts de malnutrition à cause de la guerre.[44] Durant la période qui mena au second conflit mondial, le fait qu'un si grand nombre d'Allemands ait connu la famine durant la Grande Guerre était au cœur des préoccupations d'Hitler et de ses desseins de domination mondiale.[45] La crainte de voir rejouer la défaite de l'Allemagne à l'issue de la Première Guerre mondiale et le projet de conquérir un nouvel espace vital pour les Allemands, le Lebensraum, convainquirent les Nazis de s'appuyer sur le ministère de l'Alimentation et de l'Agriculture du Reich pour élaborer une politique remédiant à la pénurie alimentaire et au rationnement qui devait assurer la victoire des Nazis.[46] Alors qu'au début de la guerre la priorité était d'augmenter la production alimentaire en Allemagne et dans les territoires occupés, ainsi que de rationner les civils et les soldats allemands, le ministère était également responsable des décisions concernant l'apport calorique destiné aux victimes de l'Holocauste dans les camps de concentration ainsi que dans les camps de prisonniers de guerre.[47] Les victimes des Nazis se voyaient octroyer de 184 à 845 calories par jour, soit un régime de restriction alimentaire extrêmement sévère.[48]

Dès 1941, il fut évident que pour assurer la victoire des Nazis contre l'Armée Rouge et atteindre la domination mondiale, la Wehrmacht (l'armée allemande) aurait besoin d'un approvisionnement en vivres que l'Allemagne seule n'était pas en mesure de produire.[49] Les calculs établis par les Nazis indiquaient que chacun des 9,5 millions d'hommes dans les troupes d'occupation allemande aurait besoin d'un apport de 3000 calories par jour afin de poursuivre ses activités militaires.[50] Dès 1943, la Wehrmacht consommait donc 40% des céréales et 62% de la viande disponibles dans le Reich, ce qui entraîna des pénuries de nourriture pour la population civile en Allemagne.[51] La question alimentaire était devenue la plus efficace des armes de guerre.

---

43. *Id. See also,* Alex De Waal, *supra* note 17, at 74; Gesine Gerhard, "Food and Genocide: Nazi Agrarian Politics in the Occupied Territories of the Soviet Union," *Contemporary European History* 18, 45–65.

44. De Waal, *supra* note 17.

45. *Id.* at 75.

46. *Id.* at 101.

47. Collingham, *supra* note 31, at 4–5.

48. *Id.*

49. *Id.* at 179–180.

50. *Id.* at 180.

51. *Id.*

Motivés par la crainte que l'Allemagne ne connaisse une défaite aussi cuisante que celle de la Première Guerre mondiale, les Nazis élaborèrent un plan qui devait assurer la défaite de l'Armée Rouge tout en assurant l'approvisionnement en vivres des Allemands pour toute la durée de la guerre.[52] De mars à mai 1941, une série de réunions eut lieu entre Herbert Backe, auteur du Plan de la faim, Hermann Göring, Plénipotentiaire du Plan de quatre ans et commandant suprême de la Luftwaffe (force aérienne allemande), Adolf Hitler et d'autres dirigeants nazis de haut-rang concernant le Plan de quatre ans du parti Nazi pour la victoire.[53] Cet entretien donna lieu à un plan destiné à affamer trente millions de « bouches inutiles » en Union Soviétique.[54] Le Plan de la faim avait pour but de catégoriser les zones de production alimentaire comme régions excédentaires ou régions déficitaires en Union Soviétique.[55] Les régions excédentaires, en particulier l'Ukraine, connue comme le grenier à blé de l'Union Soviétique, de même que le sud de la Russie et la région du Caucase, devaient être prises par la Wehrmacht afin de pouvoir envoyer 8,7 millions de tonnes d'excédents alimentaires en Allemagne, alors que les régions déficitaires, les grands centres urbains comme Moscou situés dans le nord et dans le centre de la Russie, qui avaient besoin de ravitaillement, furent coupées de toutes sources d'approvisionnement dans un but d'extermination de la population civile.[56] Si cette politique avait eu le succès escompté, elle aurait entraîné la famine de trente millions de slaves et de juifs en Union Soviétique.[57]

En mai 1941, les Nazis organisèrent la conférence de Wannsee dans la commune lacustre du même nom aux alentours de Berlin. A l'issue de cette conférence, un document d'une vingtaine de pages décrivant les grandes orientations de politique économique pour l'Organisation économique des régions occupées de l'Est qui décrivait le Plan de faim fut distribué aux hauts responsables nazis.[58] Il y figurait ce qui suit :

> La population de ces territoires, en particulier la population urbaine devra faire face à la plus terrible des famines...Des dizaines de millions de personnes dans ce territoire deviendront

---

52. De Waal, *supra* note 17, at 102; Gerhard, *supra* note 43, at 46–47.
53. Alex J. Kay, *Exploitation, Resettlement, Mass Murder: Political and Economic Planning for German Occupation Policy in the Soviet Union, 1940–1941*, 47–67 (2011 e-book).
54. De Waal, *supra* note 17, at 102; Gerhard, *supra* note 43, at 46.
55. Gerhard, *supra* note 43, at 56–57.
56. *Id. See also*, Kay, *supra* note 53, at 127.
57. De Waal, *supra* note 17, at 102–3.
58. Gerhard, *supra* note 43, at 58.

inutiles et mourront ou devront émigrer en Sibérie. Les tentatives d'y réduire la population à la mort par la famine en effectuant la saisie de la production agricole excédentaire provenant de la région des terres noires ne peuvent se faire qu'au détriment de l'approvisionnement de l'Europe. Ces excédents de production empêchent l'Allemagne de tenir jusqu'à la fin de la guerre, ils empêchent l'Allemagne et l'Europe de résister au blocus.[59]

Leur plan d'action ainsi officialisé, les Nazis déclenchèrent le pire crime de famine intentionnelle de l'histoire de l'humanité.[60]

Les Nazis mirent en œuvre le Plan de la faim sous couvert de l'Opération Barbarossa, soit l'invasion de l'Union Soviétique par les puissances de l'Axe.[61] Toutefois, les Nazis firent une erreur de calcul quant à l'ampleur de l'offensive et, par un phénomène d'usure, furent incapables de mener leur armée à la victoire contre l'Armée Rouge, cette dernière ayant réussi à épuiser la Wehrmacht en assurant des pertes constantes parmi ses soldats.[62] Les Nazis avaient sévèrement sous-estimé la difficulté qu'il y aurait à assurer la défaite de l'Armée Rouge en surnombre de 2:1 par rapport à la Wehrmacht.[63] Néanmoins, en dépit de cette erreur d'évaluation, les Nazis accomplirent en partie leur objectif décrit dans le Plan de la faim : l'Opération Barbarossa entraîna la mort d'un million de Soviétiques par la famine occasionnée au cours du Siège de Léningrad qui dura 900 jours.[64] De plus, un à deux millions de prisonniers de guerre soviétiques périrent de famine dans les camps de travail nazis.[65]

Une des raisons majeures de l'échec des objectifs principaux inscrits dans le Plan de la faim est dû au fait que les Nazis ont sous-estimé la difficulté et le temps nécessaires pour réduire trente millions de personnes à la famine. À savoir que la famine totale entraîne la mort d'un humain de constitution moyenne en deux mois.[66] D'histoire récente, on citera en

---

59. Kay, *supra* note 53, at 135.

60. De Waal, *supra* note 17, at 15.

61. *Id.* at 102.

62. Holocaust Encyclopedia, "Invasion of the Soviet Union, June 1941, US Holocaust Memorial Museum," https://encyclopedia.ushmm.org/content/en/article/invasion-of-the-soviet-union-june-1941.

63. Reina Pennington, "Was the Russian Military a Steamroller? From World War II to Today," *War on the Rocks* (Jul. 6, 2016), https://warontherocks.com/2016/07/was-the-russian-military-a-steamroller-from-world-war-ii-to-today/.

64. Collingham, *supra* note 31, at 5.

65. *Id.* at 193; Gerhard, *supra* note 43, at 60–61.

66. Collingham, *supra* note 31, at 5–6; De Waal, *supra* note 17, at 21.

exemple le membre de l'IRA, Bobby Sands, décédé à l'issue d'une grève de la faim de soixante-six jours.[67] Cependant, les Nazis ne furent pas capable de totalement couper les vivres à l'Union Soviétique, ce qui s'explique en partie par la relative disponibilité de la nourriture au marché noir.[68] Ainsi, il fut plus long que prévu de réduire la population civile à la famine tout en tentant d'assurer la défaite de l'Armée Rouge par le combat. Le projet était trop ambitieux pour les Nazis qui finirent par battre en retraite.[69] Ainsi, le Plan de la faim Nazi dans lequel était prévue l'extermination de trente millions de personnes fit environ 4,7 millions de victimes.[70] Si l'objectif initial du Plan de la faim avait été atteint, il se serait agi de la pire atrocité jamais commise de mémoire d'humain.

En dépit du fait que 4,7 millions de personnes aient trouvé la mort par les effets du Plan de la faim, ni Herbert Backe, ni Hermann Göring, ni Walter Darré (ministre de l'Alimentation et de l'Agriculture du Reich pendant le Plan de la faim) ne furent soumis à quelconque poursuite judiciaire pour violation du droit de la guerre concernant la famine des populations civiles comme méthode de guerre, du fait que la coutume de l'époque n'interdisait pas la famine comme méthode de guerre. Néanmoins, comme il a été débattu plus haut, l'utilisation de la famine comme arme de prédilection du Plan de la faim est *malum in se*, d'une part, parce que la famine intentionnelle ne peut être justifiée moralement ou éthiquement par les principes du DIH, et d'autre part, parce qu'elle ne remplit aucune des conditions de la doctrine du double effet. Il est évident qu'elle n'obéit pas à la première, car la famine utilisée tant qu'arme ne peut être ni moralement acceptable ni moralement indifférente. Elle n'obéit pas non plus à la deuxième condition de cette doctrine, car l'intention des Nazis ne fut en aucun cas d'obtenir un bon effet, mais plutôt d'exterminer trente millions de Soviétiques afin de nourrir l'armée allemande. La troisième condition n'est pas plus respectée puisque la famine de quatre millions de personnes est un mauvais effet auquel ne préside aucune justification. Quant à la quatrième condition, elle n'est pas non plus mise en pratique puisque ce qu'on pourrait peut-être comprendre comme le « bon » effet (soit le détournement de vivres saisis en Union Soviétique pour être

---

67. *Id.*
68. Kay, *supra* note 53, at 134–35.
69. Encyclopedia Britannica Online, "Stalingrad and the German retreat, summer 1942–February 1943," https://www.britannica.com/event/World-War-II/Stalingrad-and-the-German-retreat-summer-1942-February-1943.
70. De Waal, *supra* note 17, at 104 (remarquant qu'il est impossible de connaître le nombre exact des victimes du Plan de la faim, mais acceptant le chiffre de 4,7 millions sur la base des calculs effectués par les plus éminents historiens de la période).

distribués à l'armée allemande) ne peut en rien compenser le mauvais effet qui consiste à réduire 4,7 millions de personnes à la famine. En somme, le Plan de la faim n'est pas justifié selon les principes du DIH et désobéit à la doctrine du double effet.

La guerre civile au Yémen

La guerre au Yémen est à l'origine de la pire crise humanitaire du monde contemporain.[71] La guerre civile qui a débuté en 2015 entre les rebelles Houthis et le gouvernement du Yémen a causé une famine généralisée qui a entraîné la mort de dizaines de milliers de civils. Plus de vingt millions de personnes y sont soumises à l'insécurité alimentaire et à des maladies évitables telles que le choléra et la malnutrition aiguë.[72] Depuis 2017, on estime que treize millions de Yéménites ont été reconnus à risque de famine[73] et qu'au moins 85.000 enfants sont morts de faim et de maladies liées à la famine.[74] Le Yémen était déjà au bord de la crise avant que la guerre n'éclate en 2015.

Connu pour être le pays le plus pauvre du Moyen-Orient, le Yémen comptait déjà 44% de sa population en état de sous-alimentation en 2012, dont cinq millions de personnes dépendantes de l'aide alimentaire

---

71. Remarques du Secrétaire général de la conférence des donateurs pour le Yémen, The United Nations Office at Geneva (Apr. 1, 2018), https://www.unog.ch/unog/website/news_media.nsf/(httpNewsByYear_en)/27F6CCAD7178F3E9C1258264003311FA?OpenDocument; *See also* Stephen O'Brien, Statement to the Security Council on Missions to Yemen, South Sudan, Somalia, and Kenya and an Update on the Oslo Conference on Nigeria and the Lake Chad Region, United Nations Security Council (Mar. 10, 2017) https://docs.unocha.org/sites/dms/Documents/ERC_USG_Stephen_OBrien_Statement_to_the_SecCo_on_Missions_to_Yemen_South_Sudan_Somalia_and_Kenya_and_update_on_Oslo.pdf (Le chef du Bureau de Nations Unies, Stephen O'Brien, s'adressant au Conseil de sécurité : « Nous nous trouvons à un moment critique de l'histoire. En ce début d'année, nous faisons déjà face à une des plus importantes crises humanitaires depuis la création des Nations Unies ») [hereinafter, O'Brien Statement 2017].
72. Humanitarian Aid, "Humanitarian crisis in Yemen remains the worst in the world, warns UN," *UN News* (Feb. 14, 2019), https://news.un.org/en/story/2019/02/1032811; Doctors Without Borders/Médecins Sans Frontières (MSF) a traité 143.467 cas de choléra et 23.319 cas de malnutrition entre mars 2015 et septembre 2019. *See* Médecins Sans Frontières, "Yemen: Crisis Update November 2019," https://www.doctorswithoutborders.org/what-we-do/news-stories/story/yemen-crisis-update-november-2019.
73. BBC News, "Yemen could be 'worst famine in 100 years,'" (Oct. 15, 2018), https://www.bbc.com/news/av/world-middle-east-45857729.
74. Bethan McKernan, "Yemen: up to 85,000 young children dead from starvation," *The Guardian* (Nov. 21, 2018), https://www.theguardian.com/world/2018/nov/21/yemen-young-children-dead-starvation-disease-save-the-children.

d'urgence.[75] Le manque d'eau était déjà un tel problème pour ce pays aride qu'en 2012 les experts prévoyaient la fin des ressources hydriques dès 2017.[76] Au début de l'année 2017, les Nations Unis ont déclaré que le Yémen était désormais en danger de famine imminente.[77] À savoir que la famine est décrite comme « une crise caractérisée par la faim généralisée qui entraîne une mortalité élevée durant un laps de temps donné »[78], et qui a des causes multiples dont « des facteurs structurels déterminant à la fois l'état de vulnérabilité et les faits déclencheurs de la crise."[79] Les famines peuvent être différenciées en termes de magnitude (nombre de victimes) et de sévérité (niveau d'insécurité alimentaire).[80] La sévérité de l'insécurité alimentaire consiste en cinq phases : (1) minimale, (2) stress, (3) crise, (4) urgence, (5) famine.[81] De nombreuses régions au Yémen sont actuellement décrites comme étant en phase 3, dite de crise, ou en phase 4, dite d'urgence.[82] Les lieux les plus touchés par l'insécurité alimentaire se trouvent dans les zones de conflit, à Al-Hodeïda, Sana'a, Ta'izz, Aden, ainsi que dans les villages côtiers de la Mer Rouge.

Les morts causées dans la population civile par la famine et les maladies qui y sont liées, comme le choléra, ne sont pas dues à des circonstances indépendantes de la volonté humaine.[83] Deux catégories d'évènements sont avant tout responsables des morts et des atteintes à l'intégrité humaine dues à la faim : (1) les attaques militaires sur les productions agricoles et de nourriture

---

75. Joseph Hincks, "What you need to know about the crisis in Yemen," *Time* (Nov. 3, 2016), https://time.com/4552712/yemen-war-humanitarian-crisis-famine/.

76. Frederika Whitehead, Water scarcity in Yemen: the country's forgotten conflict, *The Guardian* (Apr. 2, 2015, 5:18 a.m.), https://www.theguardian.com/global-development-professionals-network/2015/apr/02/water-scarcity-yemen-conflict; IRIN in Sana'a, "Time running out for solution to Yemen's water crisis," *The Guardian* (Aug. 27, 2912, 7:30 a.m.), https://www.theguardian.com/global-development/2012/aug/27/solution-yemen-water-crisis.

77. O'Brien Statement 2017, *supra* note 71.

78. Alex De Waal, "The end of famine? Prospects for the elimination of mass starvation by political action," *Political Geography* 62 (2018): 184, 185.

79. *Id.* at 185.

80. Paul Howe and Stephen Deveraux, "Famine Intensity and Magnitude Scales: A proposal for an instrumental definition of famine," *Disasters* 28 (2004): 353–372; Famine Early Warning Systems Network, Integrated Phase Classification, https://fews.net/IPC.

81. Famine Early Warning Systems Network, "Integrated Phase Classification," https://fews.net/IPC. Traduction en français : https://www.ipcinfo.org/fileadmin/templates/ipcinfo/Docs/IPC_Facsheet_FR.pdf

82. Famine Early Warning Systems Network, "Yemen Food Security Outlook," October 2019 to May 2020, https://fews.net/east-africa/yemen/food-security-outlook/october-2019.

83. *See generally* De Waal, *supra* note 17.

détruisant, déniant l'accès ou rendant inutilisables les biens indispensables à la survie des civils, et (2) les blocus des aéroports et ports maritimes entravant l'acheminement de l'aide humanitaire.[84] Les groupes responsables de ces atrocités incluent toutes les parties prenantes dans le conflit : les rebelles Houthis soutenus par l'Iran, le gouvernement et l'armée yéménite aussi bien que la coalition menée par l'Arabie Saoudite, l'Alliance islamique pour combattre le terrorisme (AMICT). Des attaques sur les réserves de nourriture destinées aux civils ont été documentées démontrant que les instigateurs prenaient des civils pour cible, une méthode de guerre caractérisée par la violation sans ambiguïté du jus in bello et de la tradition de la guerre juste.[85] Certaines informations incriminent le prince héritier de la couronne saoudienne, Mohammed ben Salmane, qui a autorisé l'utilisation de la famine comme méthode de guerre pour assurer la défaite des Houthis.[86]

L'un des facteurs majeurs de la famine et des maladies inhérentes à la famine au Yémen est la destruction délibérée et disproportionnée des biens indispensables à la survie de la population civile, ce qui comprend des attaques menées sur des infrastructures essentielles telles les sources d'électricité, l'arrivée en eau, les barrages d'irrigation, les infrastructures agricoles d'assistance technique et les établissements de santé. Le compte-rendu du Conseil des droits de l'homme indique que les frappes aériennes de l'AMICT ont occasionné des dommages significatifs portés aux biens de caractère civil entraînant de nombreux décès.[87] La destruction de biens indispensables à la survie dans les villes de Ta'izz et de Tihama, ainsi que sur les rives de la mer Rouge, comptent parmi les incidents les plus flagrants de cette guerre, causant la famine parmi la population.

Connu comme l'un des plus importants champs de bataille dans le conflit entre les rebelles Houthis et l'AMICT, le gouvernorat de Ta'izz a essuyé un

---

84. Martha Mundy, "The Strategies of the Coalition in the Yemen War: Aerial Bombardment and Food War," *World Peace Foundation* 11 (2018), https://sites.tufts.edu/wpf/files/2018/10/Strategies-of-Coalition-in-Yemen-War-Final-20181005-1.pdf [hereinafter Mundy].

85. *Id.* at 24.

86. Un diplomate chevronné de l'AMICT a déclaré officieusement : "Once we control them, we will feed them.", « Une fois qu'on les aura sous notre contrôle, on les nourrira ». *Id.* at 7; *See also* "Bin Salman threatens to target women and children in Yemen despite international criticism," *Middle East Monitor* (Aug. 27, 2018, 10:39 a.m.), https://www.middleeastmonitor.com/20180827-bin-salman-threatens-to-target-women-and-children-in-yemen-despite-international-criticism/.

87. UN Office of the High Commissioner on Human Rights, *Yemen: United Nations Experts point to possible war crimes by parties to the conflict* (Aug. 28, 2018), https://www.ohchr.org/EN/NewsEvents/Pages/DisplayNews.aspx?NewsID=23479.

des nombres de victimes les plus élevés de cette guerre. Dès 2014, les biens de caractère civil ont été ciblés de nombreuses fois, ce qui a entraîné la mort et le déplacement forcé de nombreux civils.[88] De plus, une variété de facteurs a fait empirer l'insécurité alimentaire à Ta'izz, entraînant la famine des civils. En effet, en résultat des combats, l'accès à la nourriture sur les marchés s'est trouvé considérablement réduit et les prix ont augmenté de manière vertigineuse, rendant la nourriture inabordable pour une grande partie de la population.[89] En outre, les attaques aériennes de l'AMICT sur les exploitations agricoles, les marchés, les offices de l'agriculture et les réseaux de transport n'ont fait qu'accroître les pénuries alimentaires.[90] En décembre 2017, les frappes aériennes ciblées de l'AMICT ont détruit le marché du quartier d'al-Ta'iziyah, causant la mort de cinquante-quatre civils et faisant trente-deux blessés.[91] Dès août 2018, soixante-quinze pour cent de la population civile de Ta'izz était frappée par l'insécurité alimentaire alors qu'au moins 85% des gens étaient dépendants de l'aide humanitaire.[92]

D'autres contrées, y compris des villages de pêcheurs, ont été ciblées au-delà des attaques sur Ta'izz. Ainsi, de mars 2015 à août 2016 furent menés de nombreux raids aériens sur des régions agricoles.[93] Sachant que le Yémen ne dispose que de 5% de terre arable, et qu'avant la guerre, seulement 3% du territoire yéménite était dédié à l'agriculture, les frappes sur les régions agricoles paraissent particulièrement monstrueuses.[94] À Tihama, les frappes sur les biens indispensables à la survie des civils n'ont pas touché les champs ou les troupeaux, mais les systèmes d'irrigation alimentés par des pompes motorisées utilisant du carburant. Conséquence directe de la guerre, dès 2011, les pénuries de carburant et la hausse des prix rendaient l'irrigation pratiquement impossible pour les exploitants agricoles.[95]

Depuis la fin des années 1970, la Banque mondiale fait des investissements dans des structures de diversion de l'eau conçues par des ingénieurs

---

88. World Peace Foundation, Accountability for Mass Starvation: Starvation in Yemen Policy Brief, World Peace Foundation, 6–7 (2019), https://sites.tufts.edu/wpf/files/2019/06/WPF-GRC-POLICY-BRIEF-Accountability-for-Starvation.-Yemen.pdf [hereinafter WPF Policy Brief].
89. *Id.* at 6–7.
90. *Id.*
91. *Id.*
92. *Id.*
93. Mundy, *supra* note 84, at 11.
94. Food and Agriculture Organization of the United Nations, "Selected Indicators," http://www.fao.org/faostat/en/?#country/249.
95. Mundy, *supra* note 84, at 13.

spécialisés. Placées sous la supervision du Bureau du développement de Tihama, la Tihama Development Authority (TDA), ces structures ont pour objectif d'assurer la répartition de l'eau vers les exploitations agricoles de la région.[96] Deux fois en août 2015 et une fois de plus en septembre, l'AMICT a mené un total de quinze raids aériens sur l'enceinte de la TDA juste en-dehors de Al-Hodeïda, et conduit trois frappes supplémentaires sur les structures collectives d'irrigation de Wadi Shibam en octobre 2015.[97] Le Yemen Data Project fait mention de deux autres attaques ciblant les infrastructures de la TDA en 2016 et de trois de plus au début de l'année 2017.[98] Par conséquent, les rendements agricoles ont baissé de 24% parmi les exploitants agricoles de Wadi Zabid et de 46% à Wadi Shibam, ce qui est dû avant tout à des pénuries d'eau d'irrigation.[99] La région de Tihama, autrefois considérée comme le grenier à blé du Yémen, a vu une baisse de la culture des sols de 51%, un déclin des rendements agricoles de 20 à 61% par hectare, et la totale disparition des fruits, des légumes et des troupeaux, entraînant l'insécurité alimentaire de 43% de la population.[100]

Quant à la pêche artisanale, elle a longtemps été une des sources majeures de la production de nourriture au Yémen. La Direction générale de la pêche dans la mer Rouge fait état de préjudices importants pour l'industrie de la pêche qui, depuis le début de la guerre jusqu'à décembre 2017, a recensé la mort de 146 pêcheurs et la destruction de 220 bateaux de pêche par les attaques aériennes perpétrées par l'AMICT en 2018.[101] Précédant le début de la guerre en 2015, le secteur des pêcheries yéménites était le deuxième secteur d'exportation du pays, constituant 2% du produit national brut du Yémen.[102]

---

96. *Id.* at 14.
97. *Id.*
98. *Id.*
99. The Water and Environment Center of San'a' University, *Food Production, Irrigation, Marketing, and Agricultural Coping Mechanisms, Tihama (Wadi Zabid and Wadi Siham), Briefing Note 2-Food Security* (FBLN, NICHE-Yem027), Flood-Based Livelihoods Network Foundation, http://spate-irrigation-org/wp-content/uploads/2018/02/Briefing-Note-2-%E2%80%93-Food-Security-pdf.
100. Flood-based Livelihoods Network Foundation, "Yemen's Burnt Granary," http://spate-irrigation.org/yemens-burnt-granary/#more-6422.
101. Taqrir 'an al-qita ' al-samaki fi-'l-bahr al-ahmar ba'd alf yaum min al-'udwan [Report on the fishing sector in the Red Sea after a thousand days of the aggression] al-Hai'ah al-'Amman li'-Masa'id al-Samakiya fi'l-Bahr al-Ahmar, 13–43 (Jan. 2018).
102. Ammar Al-Fareh, "The Impact of the War in Yemen on Artisanal Fishing of the Red Sea," *LSE Middle East Centre Report* 7 (2018), http://eprints.lse.ac.uk/91022/1/Al-Fareh_The-impact-of-war_Author.pdf.

Une autre cause majeure de la famine au Yémen est imputable aux entraves posées à l'acheminement du secours humanitaire ainsi qu'à l'instrumentalisation de cette aide, qui sont entraînées par des blocus. Les obstacles à l'acheminement de fournitures humanitaires et à la mise en œuvre d'opérations de secours démontrent que les blocus ont mis fin à la livraison de l'assistance humanitaire ou ont causé des retards de transport dans les régions affectées par la famine.

Al-Hodeïda était le gouvernorat le plus pauvre du Yémen avant le début de la guerre en 2015.[103] À cette époque, soixante pour cent de la population du Yémen touchée par la malnutrition venait d'Al-Hodeïda.[104] Il faut savoir qu'il y a trois ports importants dans le gouvernorat dont deux, Al-Hodeïda et Salif, par lesquels transite la majorité des importations de nourriture du pays. Or, le chiffre des importations commerciales a considérablement chuté depuis 2014.[105] Il y a deux autres ports au Yémen situés à Aden et à Al Moukalla auxquels il manque les infrastructures nécessaires à la réception de cargaisons alimentaires.[106] En avril 2015, l'AMICT a entamé un blocus sur les ports de la mer Rouge pour inspecter les navires de commerce afin de saisir de potentielles armes illégales destinées aux Houthis.[107] La conséquence de ce blocus qui dura seize mois fut de limiter la livraison de nourriture, de carburant et de médicaments à la population civile.[108] Le 6 novembre 2017, l'AMICT a pris des mesures de rétorsion à cause d'une attaque de missiles houthie sur Riyad en imposant un blocus total du Yémen par air, terre et mer d'une durée de seize jours, empêchant ainsi toute entrée de nourriture et de carburant dans le pays,[109] et entraînant une insécurité alimentaire accrue ainsi que des morts dues à la faim et à la malnutrition.

La guerre au Yémen est un cas bien différent de celui du Plan de la faim des Nazis. Alors que les Nazis utilisaient la famine comme arme d'extermination, l'AMICT utilise le blocus et l'attaque aérienne sur les bastions houthis. Même s'il était possible d'apporter la preuve que les tactiques de l'AMICT n'ont pas intentionnellement réduit la population à la famine ou ciblé la destruction des biens indispensables à la survie des civils, ce qui serait très difficile sur la base des éléments présentés plus haut, ces tactiques

---

103. WPF Policy Brief, *supra* note 88, at 7.
104. *Id.*
105. *Id.*
106. *Id.* at 7–8.
107. *Id.*
108. *Id.* at 8.
109. *Id.*

sont néanmoins malum in se, car leur résultat brille par son indifférence irraisonnée face à la famine des civils dans la plus parfaite violation des quatre principes du DIH. De plus, bien que les blocus et les raids aériens de l'AMICT au Yémen entendent obtenir un bon effet (en l'occurrence d'assurer la défaite des rebelles houthis et de rétablir la paix et la sécurité dans la région), le mauvais effet (soit la famine) n'est pas justifié d'après la troisième et la quatrième condition de la doctrine du double effet, car il est inadmissible d'employer un mauvais moyen pour accomplir un but louable, et l'objectif de mettre fin à la guerre, qui n'a de toute façon pas été rempli, n'est pas proportionnel aux morts de faim parmi les civils. Pour ces raisons, je me positionne en faveur d'interdictions plus strictes quant aux méthodes de guerre légales entraînant directement ou indirectement la famine.

Quatrième partie : Conclusion

Ce travail met en avant que l'utilisation de la famine comme méthode de guerre devrait être absolument interdite sous couvert du droit international, car elle est *malum in se*. D'aucuns soutiendront que le DIH et le DPI interdisent déjà la famine en tant qu'arme de guerre, mais je considère que les dispositions légales en vigueur interdisant la famine sont insuffisantes, d'une part, parce qu'elles ne sont pas appliquées et, d'autre part, parce qu'elles permettent l'existence de la famine quand elle est une conséquence indirecte de méthodes légales de guerres, tels les sièges et les blocus. Ces problèmes soulignent la nécessité d'imposer des restrictions plus importantes à ce phénomène, sous couvert du cadre législatif existant, afin d'empêcher la famine intentionnelle de jamais être le résultat acceptable d'un objectif militaire, que ce soit de manière directe ou indirecte.

Le problème de l'application des lois tient en grande partie au fait que les exemples les plus récents de famine intentionnelle au Yémen et en Syrie ne tombent pas sous le coup de la Cour pénale internationale. Sans le renvoi du Conseil de sécurité de l'ONU à la CPI, il est très improbable que les instigateurs de tels crimes utilisant la famine comme arme de guerre soient tenus responsables de leurs actes[110] parce le système judiciaire de ces états corrompus est soit incapable, soit peu enclin à entamer de quelconques poursuites judiciaires à l'encontre des coupables. Ainsi, le mieux que l'on puisse faire est de conserver les preuves de ces crimes et de les employer à bon escient dans des procès futurs de façon à ce que la communauté inter-

---

110. Graham, *supra* note 27.

nationale puisse exercer une pression notable sur les membres du Conseil de sécurité, en particulier sur ses membres permanents, le p.3 (constitué des États-Unis, de la Chine et de la Russie), les encourageant à adopter une résolution au Chapitre VII de la Charte des Nations Unies dans le but d'enquêter sur les crimes causés par la famine au Yémen et en Syrie et de recommander des poursuites contre les coupables.

Une autre manière de mettre fin à l'utilisation de la famine en tant qu'arme de guerre est d'inciter les États à faire des déclarations officielles pour condamner ce fait et pour exiger une législation ou un développement progressif du droit international imposant des restrictions à la famine comme arme de guerre. Certaines stratégies au service de cet objectif pourraient inclure la caractérisation du crime de famine en tant que norme impérative du *jus cogens* à laquelle les États ne pourraient se soustraire sous couvert des traités et conventions existants,[111] et une pression accrue sur le Conseil de sécurité afin qu'il adopte une résolution au Chapitre VII de la Charte des Nations Unies demandant la fin de l'utilisation de la famine comme arme de guerre et sa description officielle comme *malum in se*. Ces progrès constitueraient un signal fort indiquant que la famine ne pourrait plus être tolérée sous couvert du droit international.

Enfin, les spécialistes de l'éthique militaire peuvent motiver des changements dans le droit en persuadant les chefs d'État et les responsables militaires que les méthodes de guerre légales pouvant entraîner la famine, de manière directe ou indirecte, ne sont pas nécessaires à l'accomplissement d'objectifs militaires. En effet, il existe d'autres moyens pouvant présider à l'accomplissement de semblables objectifs sans entraîner les conséquences insidieuses de la souffrance des civils causée par la famine. Ainsi, un revirement de point de vue parmi les responsables militaires et les chefs d'État pourrait créer une nouvelle coutume imposant la famine comme *malum in se*, ce qui faciliterait la mise en place de restrictions légales significatives sur son utilisation en temps de guerre, mettant ainsi un terme à l'impunité des instigateurs d'actes criminels par la faim.

---

111. Le travail de la Commission du droit international sur les normes impératives du droit international général (*jus cogens*) ne mentionne pas l'interdiction de la famine dans son rapport le plus récent. Toutefois, l'interdiction s'appliquant aux crimes contre l'humanité et au génocide est intimement liée à la famine comme arme de guerre. *Voir* Int'l Law Com., Peremptory norms of general international law (*jus cogens*), Text of the draft conclusions and draft annex provisionally adopted by the Drafting Committee on first reading, (May 29, 2019), A/CN.4/L.936.

The Virtuous (Human) Soldier
A MacIntyrian Approach to Moral Education in the US Army
Thesis Summary

Nathan J. Riehl

Following nearly two decades of continuous conflict, the complexities of modern warfare have placed immense pressure on the US Army to recognize its deficiencies, construct creative solutions, and adapt in a rapidly evolving environment.[1] Among the most significant changes has been the explicit branding of the army as a profession with an official ethic meant to ground the development of soldiers into competent and committed leaders of character.[2] The army profession views this developmental process as crucial to maintaining a foundation of trust with its client—the American people. By morally educating every soldier to be a leader of character, the army better prepares them to face the multitude of ethical challenges accompanying modern warfare in the presence of multinational conditions, the geopolitical situation, and advancements in media and technology.[3] Additionally, the army's character development process plays a large part in shaping the soldier qua human, guiding an individual's decisions and actions in the other various roles they occupy within society both now and throughout the rest of their life. Therefore, the army should instill an ethical framework that not only serves soldiers on the battlefield, but also in their homes and throughout their post-military careers. In this thesis I argue that the unique nature of the army profession requires an expansion from a general moral education process aimed at developing virtuous soldiers to a more holistic moral development of humans seeking a flourishing life

---

1. The views expressed throughout this thesis are my own and do not necessarily reflect those of the US Army, the Department of Defense, or the US government.
2. US Dept. of the Army. *Army White Paper: The Army's Framework for Character Development.* Center for the Army Profession and Ethic, 2017, 2. The Army defines character as "one's true nature including identity, sense of purpose, values, virtues, morals, and conscience." Further, it is "the moral and ethical qualities that help us determine what is right and provide motivation to act accordingly."
3. US Dept. of the Army. ADP 6-22 Army Leadership and the Profession. Government Printing Office, 2019, 8-4.

while fulfilling the various roles of a soldier. I approach this task utilizing a framework initially laid out by Alasdair MacIntyre in his book, *After Virtue*. Specifically, I critique the US Army character development process utilizing two of the three logical stages in MacIntyre's development of the concept of a virtue—"practice" and "narrative."[4] As I move through the first two stages of MacIntyre's concept of a virtue, I argue that while the army's moral education process attempts something very similar to MacIntyre's framework, there are crucial gaps that prevent the proper moral development of soldiers from taking place.[5]

In the first section, I introduce the roles MacIntyre's practice and narrative order of a single human life play in the development of a virtue. More specifically, MacIntyre's account of virtues first proceeds through a stage which concerns virtues as qualities necessary to achieve the goods internal to practices, followed by a second stage which considers them as qualities contributing to the good of a whole life.[6] In considering the first stage, I argue that the army is not a singular practice, but a collection of practices, each requiring a unique set of virtues. Practices encompass a great many things including arts, sciences, games, and the making and sustaining of family life.[7] In entering a practice an individual accepts the authority of certain standards of excellence and obedience to rules that place judgement upon the inadequacy of their own performance. To enter into a practice is to accept the current state of standards realized so far in the progression of the practice itself, and to live out the good of a certain kind of life.[8] The army attempts to instill virtues it believes are necessary for professional soldiers, yet they fail to capture the uniqueness and diversity of the various soldiering roles. Currently, these soldier virtues are codified in the official Army Values of loyalty, duty, respect, selfless service, honor, integrity, and personal courage.[9]

---

4. While I believe the Army could benefit from elements within the tradition stage of MacIntyre's framework, the complexity of addressing the stage was too unwieldly given the purpose of this thesis.

5. I believe that values, like the Army Values, are what we aim for and virtues, in a MacIntyrian sense, are those values which we have successfully attained. I use both terms interchangeably here, but the difference in the context of this paper is the difference of the starting point and ending point of a successful moral education process.

6. Alasdair MacIntyre, *After Virtue*, 3rd ed. (University of Notre Dame Press, 2007), 273.

7. MacIntyre, *After Virtue*, 188.

8. MacIntyre, *After Virtue*, 190.

9. US Dept. of the Army, *ADP 6-22 Army Leadership and the Profession*, Government Printing Office, 2019, 1–2. The Army is explicit in its Army Value of "personal courage" pertaining to both physical courage as well as moral courage.

To demonstrate that the army is no longer a singular practice of soldiering, I focus on three distinct army branches in the Infantry, Signal Corps, and Civil Affairs. By highlighting the uniqueness of each branch, I argue that the army is in fact a community built around a collection of practices, much like a scientific society built around multiple scientific practices, or an orchestra built around a collection of instrumental practices.[10] Importantly, each of these practices requires a unique collection of virtues necessary to flourishing within that particular role.

In considering MacIntyre's second stage, I argue that the holistic narrative of individual soldiers and the various roles they occupy outside of the military—which are vital to proper moral deliberation—are essentially nonfactors in the moral education process of the US Army. The concept of a virtue must continue its development through the second stage of the framework, in which an individual considers their various practices and virtues within the unity of an individual life—MacIntyre's narrative. It is through narrative that an individual establishes their selfhood and recognizes that they are the subject of a history that they must own. In doing so, an individual becomes accountable for their actions and experiences. While the army acknowledges that each soldier possesses an individual narrative with unique personal values, they fail to consider their importance to the proper moral development of a soldier as a human. A soldier's personal roles, whether as a spouse, parent, citizen, or friend, are vitally important in establishing a unified individual life capable of moral reasoning. By disregarding such a crucial component in the educational process, the army attempts to set the priorities of a soldier's narrative believing that it might eliminate potential conflicts. However, conflict between personal and professional values remains inevitable and to ignore such conflict in the education process leaves soldiers ill-prepared to face ethical tension well as moral agents. While highlighting this inevitable tension, I explore three scenarios in which the Army Values can conflict with the other practices and virtues of an individual soldier.[11] Instead of attempting to eliminate ethical tension, proper moral development consists of educating soldiers on the possibility of error and of the errors to which each of them may

10. Kenneth A. Strike, "Trust, Traditions and Pluralism: Human Flourishing and Liberal Polity," in *Virtue Ethics and Moral Education*, ed. David Carr and Jan Steutel (Routledge, 1999), 239.

11. Eva Van Baarle et al, "Moral Dilemmas in a Military Context. A Case Study of a Train the Trainer Course on Military Ethics," *Journal of Moral Education* 44, no. 4 (2015): 465.

be inclined. This requires guiding soldiers in the acknowledgment of and reflection upon who they are as individuals and the various roles they may hold as spouses, parents, citizens, or friends.[12] The moral education of soldiers in the virtues of a practice requires the ability to demonstrate not only how they will serve in the good soldier life, but also how they may contribute to life as a whole.

Ultimately, I argue that the unique nature of the army profession requires an expansion from a general moral education process aimed at developing virtuous soldiers to one which aims to morally develop soldiers holistically as humans seeking a flourishing life in their role as a soldier. In recognizing my argument as a significant departure from the current US Army character development process, I consider two possible objections. First, an objection that asks whether it is an army's responsibility to morally develop its force beyond their roles as soldiers. Second, an objection that asks whether the US Army could feasibly embrace a MacIntyrian approach. To both, I argue yes, as the US Army's responsibility to defend the nation and the moral development of its soldiers are intertwined now more than ever. The immense moral responsibility that young and increasingly autonomous volunteer soldiers face today requires the US Army to accept the responsibility, and I offer some practical steps for addressing practice and narrative in the soldier moral education process.

Works Cited

MacIntyre, Alasdair. After Virtue. 3rd ed., University of Notre Dame Press, 2007.
———. *Ethics in the Conflicts of Modernity: An Essay on Desire, Practical Reasoning, and Narrative.* Cambridge University Press, 2016.
Strike, Kenneth A. "Trust, Traditions and Pluralism: Human Flourishing and Liberal Polity." In *Virtue Ethics and Moral Education*, edited by David Carr and Jan Steutel, 231-244. Routledge, 1999.
Van Baarle, Eva, et al. "Moral Dilemmas in a Military Context. A Case Study of a Train the Trainer Course on Military Ethics." *Journal of Moral Education* 44, no. 4 (2015): 457-478.
US Dept. of the Army. ADP 6-22 Army Leadership and the Profession. Government Printing Office, 2019.
US Dept. of the Army. Army White Paper: The Army's Framework for Character Development. Center for the Army Profession and Ethic, 2017.

---

12. Alasdair MacIntyre, *Ethics in the Conflicts of Modernity: An Essay on Desire, Practical Reasoning, and Narrative* (Cambridge University Press, 2016), 191.

El soldado (humano) virtuoso
Un enfoque macintyriano hacia la educación moral en el ejército de Estados Unidos
Resumen de tesis

Nathan J. Riehl

Después de casi dos décadas de incesante conflicto, las complejidades de la guerra moderna han ejercido una enorme presión sobre el ejército estadounidense para que reconozca sus deficiencias, elabore soluciones creativas y se adapte en un entorno de rápida evolución.[1] Uno de los cambios más significativos ha sido promocionar de manera explícita al ejército como una profesión que posee una ética oficial destinada a cimentar el desarrollo de soldados como líderes de carácter, competentes y comprometidos.[2] La profesión militar considera este proceso de desarrollo como crucial para mantener una base de confianza con su cliente: el pueblo estadounidense. Al educar moralmente a cada soldado para que sea un líder de carácter, el ejército los prepara de mejor manera para enfrentar el sinnúmero de desafíos éticos inherentes a la guerra moderna ante la presencia de las condiciones multinacionales, la situación geopolítica y los avances de los medios de comunicación y de la tecnología.[3] Así mismo, el proceso de forjar el carácter militar juega un papel trascendental en la formación del soldado como ser humano, guiando las decisiones y las acciones del individuo en los diversos roles que desempeña dentro de la sociedad, tanto en el presente como en el resto de su vida. Por lo tanto, el ejército debe inculcar un marco de referencia ético que no solo apoye a los soldados en el campo de batalla, sino también en sus hogares y

---

1. Las opiniones expresadas a lo largo de esta tesis son mías y no reflejan necesariamente las del ejército estadounidense, del Departamento de Defensa o del gobierno de los EE.UU.
2. US Dept. of the Army. *Army White Paper: The Army's Framework for Character Development* [Libro blanco del ejército: El marco del ejército para el desarrollo del carácter]. Center for the Army Profession and Ethic, 2017, 2. El ejército define el término carácter como "la verdadera naturaleza de uno mismo, incluyendo la identidad, el sentido del propósito, los valores, las virtudes, la moral y la conciencia". Además, son "las cualidades morales y éticas las que nos ayudan a determinar lo que es correcto y nos motivan a actuar en consecuencia".
3. US Dept. of the Army. ADP 6-22 *Army Leadership and the Profession* [Liderazgo del ejército y la profesión]. Government Printing Office, 2019, 8-4.

durante su carrera post-militar. En la presente tesis, sostengo que la singular naturaleza de la profesión militar precisa de la expansión de un proceso de educación moral general dirigido a formar soldados virtuosos, a un desarrollo moral más integral de seres humanos que buscan una vida plena a la vez que cumplen con los diversos roles de un soldado. Abordo este planteamiento utilizando un marco teórico que fue propuesto inicialmente por Alasdair MacIntyre en su libro Tras la virtud. De manera específica, realizo una crítica del proceso de desarrollo del carácter del ejército estadounidense utilizando dos de las tres fases lógicas de MacIntyre en el desarrollo del concepto de una virtud: "práctica" y "narrativa".[4] A medida que analizo las dos primeras fases de MacIntyre sobre el concepto de una virtud sostengo que, si bien el proceso de educación moral militar intenta lograr algo muy similar al marco teórico de MacIntyre, existen vacíos cruciales que impiden que se produzca el desarrollo moral adecuado de los soldados.[5]

En la primera sección expongo los roles que juegan la práctica y el orden narrativo macintyrianos de una sola vida humana en el desarrollo de una virtud. La postura de las virtudes de MacIntyre pasa más concretamente, primero por una fase que considera las virtudes como cualidades necesarias para alcanzar los bienes internos de las prácticas, seguida de una segunda fase que las considera como cualidades que contribuyen al beneficio de una vida plena.[6] Al considerar la primera fase, sostengo que el ejército no es una sola práctica, sino un conjunto de prácticas, cada una de las cuales requiere de un conjunto de virtudes único. Las prácticas abarcan una gran cantidad de elementos que incluyen las artes, las ciencias, los juegos y la creación y la subsistencia de la vida familiar.[7] Al ingresar en una práctica, el individuo acepta la autoridad de ciertos estándares de excelencia y la obediencia de reglas que sopesan la deficiencia de su propio desempeño. Ingresar en una práctica significa la aceptación del estado actual de los estándares establecidos hasta hoy en el avance de la práctica misma y disfrutar del beneficio de cierto

---

4. Aunque considero que el ejército podría beneficiarse de los elementos contemplados dentro de la fase tradicional del marco de MacIntyre, la complejidad de abordarla resultaba demasiado intrincada para los fines de la presente tesis.

5. Considero que los valores, al igual que los Valores del Ejército, son lo que buscamos y en un sentido macintyriano, las virtudes son los valores que hemos logrado con éxito. Aquí utilizo ambos términos indistintamente, sin embargo, en el contexto de este documento se distinguen por la diferencia entre el punto de partida y el punto de llegada de un proceso de educación moral que ha tenido éxito.

6. Alasdair MacIntyre, *After Virtue* [Tras la virtud], 3rd ed. (University of Notre Dame Press, 2007), 273.

7. MacIntyre, *After Virtue*, 188.

tipo de vida.[8] El ejército intenta inculcar aquellas virtudes que considera necesarias para los soldados profesionales. Sin embargo, no logra captar la singularidad y diversidad de los múltiples roles que aquellos desempeñan. Estas virtudes del soldado se encuentran actualmente tipificadas en los Valores oficiales de lealtad, deber, respeto, servicio desinteresado, honor, integridad y valentía personal del Ejército[9] Para probar que el ejército ya no es una práctica exclusiva de la milicia, me concentro en tres diferentes ramas del ejército: la Infantería, el Cuerpo de Señales y el de Asuntos Civiles. Al destacar la singularidad de cada rama, sostengo que el ejército constituye, de hecho, una comunidad fundada en torno a un conjunto de prácticas muy similares a las de una sociedad científica cimentada en torno a múltiples prácticas científicas o las de una orquesta formada en torno a un conjunto de prácticas instrumentales.[10] Cabe destacar que cada una de estas prácticas precisa de un singular conjunto de virtudes necesario para desarrollarse dentro de ese rol en particular.

Con respecto a la segunda fase de MacIntyre, sostengo que la narrativa holística de los soldados en lo individual y los diversos roles que desempeñan fuera del ejército, los cuales son vitales para una adecuada ponderación moral, no son básicamente, factores en el proceso de educación moral del ejército estadounidense. El concepto de virtud debe continuar desarrollándose a través de la segunda fase del marco en la que un individuo considere sus diversas prácticas y virtudes dentro de la unidad de una vida individual, o sea, la narrativa de MacIntyre. Es a través de la narrativa que un individuo establece su propio ser y reconoce que es el sujeto de una historia que debe pertenecerle. Y al hacerlo, se responsabiliza de sus acciones y experiencias. Si bien el ejército reconoce que todo soldado posee una narrativa individual con valores personales únicos, se equivoca al no considerar su importancia con respecto al adecuado desarrollo moral de un soldado como ser humano. Los roles personales de un soldado, ya sea como cónyuge, padre, ciudadano o amigo, son de vital importancia para establecer una vida personal unificada apta para un razonamiento moral. Al ignorar dicho componente fundamen-

---

8. MacIntyre, *After Virtue*, 190.

9. US Dept. of the Army, *ADP 6-22 Army Leadership and the Profession* [Liderazgo del ejército y la profesión], Government Printing Office, 2019, 1–2. El Ejército es explícito en cuanto al Valor del Ejército sobre "valor personal", el cual se refiere tanto a la valentía física como a la moral.

10. Kenneth A. Strike, "Trust, Traditions and Pluralism: Human Flourishing and Liberal Polity," [Confianza, tradiciones y pluralismo: el florecimiento humano y política liberal] en *Virtue Ethics and Moral Education*, ed. David Carr and Jan Steutel (Routledge, 1999), 239.

tal en el proceso educativo, el ejército intenta establecer las prioridades de la narrativa de un soldado bajo la creencia de con esto se podrían eliminar conflictos potenciales. Sin embargo, el conflicto entre los valores personales y los profesionales sigue siendo inevitable e ignorar dicho conflicto en el proceso educativo impide que los soldados se preparen adecuadamente para enfrentar como sujetos morales, las tensiones éticas. Al mismo tiempo que destaco esta inevitable tensión, analizo tres situaciones en las que los Valores del Ejército pueden entrar en conflicto con las demás prácticas y virtudes de un soldado en lo individual.[11] En lugar de tratar de eliminar la tensión ética, el desarrollo moral adecuado consiste en educar a los soldados con respecto a la posibilidad de error y de los errores que cada uno de ellos pudiera cometer. Lo anterior precisa de orientar a los soldados para que reconozcan y reflexionen sobre quiénes son como individuos y sobre los diversos roles que pueden llegar a desempeñar como cónyuges, padres, ciudadanos o amigos.[12] La educación moral de los soldados en cuanto a las virtudes de una práctica, requiere de la capacidad para demostrar, no sólo cómo podrán prestar servicio en su vida de buen soldado, sino también cómo podrían contribuir a la vida en su conjunto.

Por último, sostengo que la singular naturaleza de la profesión militar precisa de la expansión de un proceso de educación moral en general, dirigido al desarrollo de soldados virtuosos, a otro que tenga como objetivo el desarrollo moral de los soldados de manera integral, como seres humanos que buscan una vida próspera en su rol de soldados. Consciente de que mi argumento se aparta de manera significativa del actual proceso de desarrollo del carácter del ejército estadounidense, planteo dos posibles objeciones. Primero, una objeción que cuestiona si es responsabilidad de un ejército desarrollar moralmente a sus conscriptos más allá de su función como soldados. Segundo, una objeción que cuestiona si el ejército estadounidense podría adoptar un enfoque macintyriano. En ambos casos sostengo que sí, puesto que hoy más que nunca se entrelazan la responsabilidad del ejército estadounidense de defender la nación y el desarrollo moral de sus soldados. La enorme responsabilidad moral que hoy enfrentan los jóvenes y los cada vez más autónomos soldados voluntarios exige que el ejército estadounidense

---

11. Eva Van Baarle et al, "Moral Dilemmas in a Military Context. A Case Study of a Train the Trainer Course on Military Ethics," [Dilemas morales en un contexto militar. Un caso de estudio de un curso de formación para formadores de ética militar] *Journal of Moral Education* 44, no. 4 (2015): 465.
12. Alasdair MacIntyre, *Ethics in the Conflicts of Modernity: An Essay on Desire, Practical Reasoning, and Narrative* [Ética en los conflictos de la modernidad: Sobre el deseo, el razonamiento práctico y la narrativa] (Cambridge University Press, 2016), 191.

acepte esa responsabilidad. Presento, asimismo, algunas medidas prácticas para abordar la práctica y la narrativa del proceso de educación moral de los soldados.

Obras citadas

MacIntyre, Alasdair. *After Virtue*. 3rd ed., University of Notre Dame Press, 2007.

———. *Ethics in the Conflicts of Modernity: An Essay on Desire, Practical Reasoning, and Narrative*. Cambridge University Press, 2016.

Strike, Kenneth A. "Trust, Traditions and Pluralism: Human Flourishing and Liberal Polity." In *Virtue Ethics and Moral Education*, edited by David Carr and Jan Steutel, 231-244. Routledge, 1999.

Van Baarle, Eva, et al. "Moral Dilemmas in a Military Context. A Case Study of a Train the Trainer Course on Military Ethics." *Journal of Moral Education* 44, no. 4 (2015): 457-478.

US Dept. of the Army. *ADP 6-22 Army Leadership and the Profession*. Government Printing Office, 2019.

US Dept. of the Army. *Army White Paper: The Army's Framework for Character Development*. Center for the Army Profession and Ethic, 2017.

Un soldat vertueux (et humain)
Pour une méthode d'éducation morale MacIntyrienne dans l'armée américaine
Résumé de la thèse

Nathan J. Riehl

A l'issue de presque deux décennies de conflit continu, les complexités de la guerre moderne ont su exercer une énorme pression sur l'armée américaine la contraignant à faire face à ses lacunes, à établir des solutions créatives pour y remédier et à s'adapter à un environnement en constante évolution.[1] Parmi les changements les plus significatifs, l'image de marque savamment ménagée d'une armée de métier, dorénavant dotée d'une déontologie officielle, censée assurer la formation de soldats de caractère qui se distinguent par leurs compétences et par la force de leur engagement.[2] La profession voit en ce processus un moyen essentiel de garder la confiance de sa clientèle, à savoir le peuple américain. En assurant une éducation morale à tous les soldats pour en faire des leaders de caractère, l'armée prépare mieux ses troupes à une multitude de défis éthiques associés à la guerre moderne dans certaines conditions multilatérales, selon une situation géopolitique donnée et compte tenu des avancées des médias et des nouvelles technologies.[3] De plus, la construction d'une identité morale joue un rôle majeur dans la formation du soldat en tant qu'humain en orientant les décisions et les actions individuelles de chacun dans ses rôles au sein de la société ainsi qu'à travers les étapes consécutives de sa vie. Dans cette optique, l'armée devrait établir un cadre éthique qui soit utile aux soldats sur le champ de bataille mais également dans leur vie

---

1. Les opinions exprimées dans ce mémoire sont personnelles et ne reflètent pas nécessairement celles de l'armée américaine, du département de la défense ou du gouvernement américain.
2. US Dept. of the Army. *Army White Paper: The Army's Framework for Character Development.* Center for the Army Profession and Ethic, 2017, 2. L'armée définit la notion de caractère en tant que « la nature profonde d'un individu comprenant identité, valeurs personnelles, morale et conscience ». De plus, ce sont « les qualités morales et éthiques qui nous aident à déterminer ce qui est juste en nous donnant la motivation d'agir en conséquence ».
3. US Dept. of the Army. ADP 6-22 *Army Leadership and the Profession.* Government Printing Office, 2019, 8-4.

courante et dans leur carrière au sortir des rangs de l'armée. Dans ce mémoire, je soutiens que la nature particulière de l'armée de métier justifie qu'une éducation fondée sur le socle d'une morale traditionnelle destinée à faire des soldats vertueux soit enrichie d'une philosophie morale holistique destinée à des humains désireux d'une existence épanouissante associée à leurs rôles divers, dont en tant que soldat. J'envisage cette tâche en recourant à un cadre de pensée proposé par Alasdair MacIntyre dans son ouvrage, After Virtue (trad. Après la vertu). J'entends précisément faire la critique du processus actuel de développement de l'identité morale au sein de l'armée en fondant mon argumentation sur deux des trois stades logiques du développement du concept de vertu selon MacIntyre : la concrétisation des biens propres à certains types d'activités humaines (la pratique) et son articulation narrative (le discours).[4] À travers leur description, je soutiens qu'en dépit des tentatives d'éducation morale de l'armée, somme toute assez semblables au cadre de pensée défini par MacIntyre, il subsiste des lacunes qui viennent entraver le développement moral des soldats.[5]

La première partie de ce mémoire est dédiée au rôle que jouent dans le développement d'une vertu la pratique et l'ordre narratif de MacIntyre observés au sein d'une seule vie humaine. Plus spécifiquement, la description des vertus selon lui passe d'abord par le premier stade où celles-ci sont perçues en tant que qualités nécessaires à la concrétisation des biens propres à certaines activités humaines, suivi d'un deuxième stade dans lequel les vertus sont vues comme des qualités contribuant à la qualité de toute une vie.[6] Concernant le premier stade, je défends l'idée que l'armée n'est non pas constituée d'une, mais de multiples pratiques singulières, chacune dépendant d'une association unique de certaines vertus. Ces pratiques peuvent englober arts, sciences, jeux, ainsi que l'élaboration et le maintien de la vie familiale.[7] En adhérant à une concrétisation possible, un individu accepte de se plier à l'autorité de certains standards d'excellence et de respect des règles qui sanctionnent l'inadéquation de leur qualité d'exécution. Adhérer à une

---

4. Quoique l'armée puisse à mon sens s'inspirer d'éléments inclus dans le troisième stade de la vertu défini par MacIntyre (soit la tradition morale historique), la complexité d'une référence à ce volet était trop étendue étant donné les limites du champ d'investigation de ce mémoire.

5. Je crois que les valeurs, comme celles de l'armée, sont liées à nos buts et que les vertus, au sens MacIntyrian du terme, sont des valeurs qui ont été atteintes. J'emploie ici ces termes dans le même sens, à une différence près ayant trait aux limites, en tant que point de départ et point d'arrivée, d'un processus d'éducation morale convaincant.

6. Alasdair MacIntyre, *After Virtue*, 3rd ed. (University of Notre Dame Press, 2007), 273.

7. MacIntyre, *After Virtue*, 188.

pratique revient à accepter les standards actuels entrant en ligne de compte dans la progression de cette pratique même, et à profiter des avantages du style de vie choisi.[8] Les tentatives promues par l'armée afin d'instiller des vertus qu'elle croit nécessaires aux soldats de métier ne parviennent pas à saisir la singularité et la diversité des rôles dans la profession. Les valeurs nécessaires aux soldats sont actuellement codifiées dans les sept principes de base officiels que sont la loyauté, le devoir, le respect, le service altruiste, l'honneur, l'intégrité et le courage.[9] Afin de faire la preuve que l'armée ne propose plus une seule et unique façon d'être soldat, je place l'accent sur trois branches distinctes, l'Infanterie, le Corps des transmissions et le Bureau des affaires civiles. En soulignant le caractère unique de chaque corps de l'armée, je soutiens que celle-ci est en fait une communauté édifiée autour de pratiques, comme une société scientifique construite autour d'une multiplicité de pratiques scientifiques, ou un orchestre édifié autour d'un ensemble de pratiques musicales.[10] De manière plus importante, chacune de ces pratiques requiert un ensemble unique de vertus nécessaires à l'épanouissement individuel dans un rôle donné.

A propos du deuxième stade de la théorie de MacIntyre, je défends l'idée qu'une narration globale produite par les soldats, de même que les rôles variés qu'ils occupent dans la vie civile, sont considérés, pour la majeure partie, comme des facteurs négligeables dans le processus d'éducation morale au sein de l'armée américaine alors qu'ils sont essentiels à une délibération morale adéquate. Le concept de vertu doit continuer à se développer au cours du deuxième stade de ce cadre de pensée, dans lequel un individu considère ses pratiques variées et ses vertus au sein de l'unité d'une vie personnelle : tel est le discours narratif décrit par MacIntyre. C'est à travers le discours narratif que l'individu établit une conscience de soi en reconnaissant qu'il est le sujet d'une histoire qu'il doit prendre en charge. Ce faisant, cet individu devient alors responsable de ses actions et de ses expériences. Toutefois, alors que l'armée prend en compte la narration individuelle de chaque soldat dans l'unicité de ses valeurs personnelles, elle peine à prendre en considération l'importance de cette narration dans le développement moral d'un soldat

---

8. MacIntyre, *After Virtue*, 190.
9. US Dept. of the Army, *ADP 6-22 Army Leadership and the Profession*, Government Printing Office, 2019, 1–2. L'armée est explicite dans le principe fondateur de « courage personnel » ce qui entend à la fois courage physique et courage moral.
10. Kenneth A. Strike, "Trust, Traditions and Pluralism: Human Flourishing and Liberal Polity," in *Virtue Ethics and Moral Education*, ed. David Carr and Jan Steutel (Routledge, 1999), 239.

en tant qu'humain. Or, les rôles individuels d'un soldat en tant qu'époux, parent, citoyen ou ami sont d'une importance cruciale dans la construction d'une vie personnelle cohérente qui soit capable de raison morale. En mettant à l'écart une composante si essentielle du processus éducatif, l'armée tente de ne donner la primauté qu'à certains aspects du discours narratif du soldat, espérant ainsi pouvoir éviter de potentiels conflits. Toutefois, le conflit entre valeurs personnelles et professionnelles reste inévitable et l'évincer du processus éducatif prépare mal les soldats à leur rôle d'agent moral quand ils se trouvent en présence de tensions éthiques. En soulignant cette inévitable tension, j'évoque trois scénarios dans lesquels les principes de base de l'armée peuvent entrer en conflit avec les autres pratiques et vertus du soldat.[11] Au lieu de tenter d'éliminer les tensions éthiques, un développement moral approprié consiste à éduquer les soldats à la possibilité de faire des erreurs ainsi qu'aux erreurs auxquelles chacun d'entre eux pourrait être enclin. Cela implique que les soldats soient guidés dans la confirmation de leur identité en tant qu'individus, ainsi que dans la réflexion au sujet de cette identité, et quant aux rôles variés qu'ils sont appelés à tenir en tant qu'époux, parents, citoyens ou amis.[12] L'éducation morale des soldats dans les vertus d'une pratique requiert l'habilité de démontrer les bénéfices de ces vertus dans la vie du bon soldat, mais aussi la manière dont celles-ci s'appliquent à l'existence en général.

En somme, je défends l'idée que le caractère unique de l'armée de métier mérite un glissement de l'éducation morale générale en place, censée former des soldats vertueux, vers un système ayant pour but de promouvoir une conception holistique du développement moral appliquée à des humains prétendant à une vie épanouissante dans leur rôle de soldat. Tout en reconnaissant l'écart significatif entre ma prise de position et celle qui sous-tend le processus de développement moral ayant cours dans l'armée américaine, je me dois de considérer deux objections. La première consiste à s'interroger sur le fait qu'il incombe ou pas à l'armée de prendre en charge l'éducation morale de ses troupes au-delà de leur rôle en tant que soldats. La seconde pose la question de savoir s'il serait faisable pour l'armée américaine d'envisager une approche macintyrienne de l'enseignement moral. En réponse à ces deux objections possibles, je soutiens que oui, car il est de la responsabilité de l'armée que de défendre la nation, le développement moral de ses soldats

11. Eva Van Baarle et al, "Moral Dilemmas in a Military Context. A Case Study of a Train the Trainer Course on Military Ethics," *Journal of Moral Education* 44, no. 4 (2015): 465.
12. Alasdair MacIntyre, *Ethics in the Conflicts of Modernity: An Essay on Desire, Practical Reasoning, and Narrative* (Cambridge University Press, 2016), 191.

y étant plus que jamais lié. L'immense responsabilité morale incombant à des engagés volontaires jeunes et de plus en plus autonomes requiert de l'armée qu'elle relève ce défi. C'est dans cette optique que je propose des solutions concrètes incluant pratique et discours narratif dans le processus d'éducation morale des soldats.

Bibliographie (en anglais) :

MacIntyre, Alasdair. *After Virtue*. 3rd ed., University of Notre Dame Press, 2007.
———. *Ethics in the Conflicts of Modernity: An Essay on Desire, Practical Reasoning, and Narrative*. Cambridge University Press, 2016.
Strike, Kenneth A. "Trust, Traditions and Pluralism: Human Flourishing and Liberal Polity." In *Virtue Ethics and Moral Education*, edited by David Carr and Jan Steutel, 231-244. Routledge, 1999.
Van Baarle, Eva, et al. "Moral Dilemmas in a Military Context. A Case Study of a Train the Trainer Course on Military Ethics." *Journal of Moral Education* 44, no. 4 (2015): 457-478.
US Dept. of the Army. *ADP 6-22 Army Leadership and the Profession*. Government Printing Office, 2019.
US Dept. of the Army. *Army White Paper: The Army's Framework for Character Development*. Center for the Army Profession and Ethic, 2017.

Artificial Intelligence as Clinician
An Argument for Ethical use of Future Technology in a
Medical Setting

Sara Gaines

In today's world, science fiction has become reality. The presence of artificial intelligence (AI) in societies around the world continues to grow, from pocket devices to globalized software. One field in particular, medicine, has taken careful note of the ways in which these technologies have been implemented and what lies on the horizon. It is no surprise that AI technologies will be implemented further into a healthcare setting, and with increased implementation comes increased concern over the ethics of using AI. As the technology has advanced, ethical concerns have always been present, but one area in particular will soon need to be at the center of these conversations—that of the patient-clinician relationship. The development and application of future technologies may place an AI in the role of medical decision-maker, thereby potentially influencing the patient-clinician relationship. A version of this technology, what I refer to as frontline AI clinicians, can be implemented in an ethical manner by following two criteria. First, frontline AI clinicians should be utilized in environments where the use of AI relieves a strain on the hospital system and allows for increased access to healthcare. Secondly, such technologies should be implemented in environments where patients have demonstrated an ability to connect on a personal level with AI technologies. In the United States, there is one hospital system that would be able to implement AI as a frontline clinician while adhering to these criteria: the Veterans Health Administration.

It is impossible not to consider the future applications of AI in medicine, given how society has already embraced AI. The Oxford English Dictionary defines *artificial intelligence* as "the theory and development of computer systems able to perform tasks that normally require human intelligence."[1]

---

1. Oxford English Dictionary Online, s.v. "artificial intelligence," November 2019. Oxford: Oxford University Press. https://www.oed.com/view/Entry/271625?redirectedFrom=artificial+intelligence#eid.

Under this definition, many technologies people use on a day-to-day basis indicate how entwined AI is with people's lives around the world. The phones we carry in our pockets are capable of quickly searching for not only the nearest place to eat with the highest ratings but can also tell you how to get there. Each of us has searched for an item online, only to see that product advertised to us across social media platforms and websites far removed from the original search. Finding new music is easier than ever, with streaming services offering new suggestions every day. These are only a few examples of AI that have easily integrated into daily life, but as the technology progresses, the presence of AI will only continue to grow. However, to examine the impact of the integration of future technologies not just in day-to-day activities, but specifically in a healthcare setting, more clarity than a dictionary definition of AI is required.

To further clarify between tasks performed by a human and technology "able to perform tasks that normally require human intelligence," AI has advanced to a stage where it can be discussed in terms of Weak AI and Strong AI. AI technologies considered to fall in the Weak AI category are those that are structured around a single human ability.[2] For example, probabilistic reasoning and visual perception. On the other hand, Strong AI covers hypothetical technologies considered to be equal to human intelligence, or even superhuman in terms of ability to execute intelligent tasks.[3] Strong AI technologies would be those that can understand symbolism, manage social settings, or have ideological thought processes of their own. In many ways, this division is synonymous with current technologies (weak) and future technologies (strong). However, this division is not binary, but exists on a scale. There are many technologies pushing the boundaries further from search algorithms or programs designed to find the next song for your playlist and toward what was once, and still in many ways, only considered possible in science fiction. Many of the ideas of AI in science fiction that focus on Strong AI technologies and how they are portrayed can and have greatly influenced AI's perception in a society. Depending on how AI is portrayed in these fictional examples, it can either harm or help how humans interact with developing technologies.

---

2. Stuart J. Russell and Peter Norvig, *Artificial Intelligence a Modern Approach* (Boston: Pearson, 2016)
3. Erik Brynjolfsson and Andrew McAfee, *The Second Machine Age: Work, Progress, and Prosperity in a Time of Brilliant Technologies* (Vancouver, BC: Langara College, 2018).

While certainly not true everywhere in the world, the United States has a very suspect view of AI technologies. Theoretical AI capable of thinking for itself has been largely portrayed as a villain in American culture. Fears of AI in the Western world were documented well before the average person began to interact with AI on a daily basis. Isaac Asimov published *I, Robot*, his collection of short stories about AI-equipped robotics and how they interact with the world around them, in 1950. Within these short stories are the famous Three Laws of Robotics:

1. A robot may not injure a human being or, through inaction, allow a human being to come to harm.
2. A robot must obey the orders given it by human beings except where such orders would conflict with the First Law.
3. A robot must protect its own existence as long as such protection does not conflict with the First or Second Laws.[4]

These laws, while adjusted and expanded upon by authors, including Asimov himself, throughout the following decades have largely influenced not just science fiction, but also the field of Artificial Intelligence ethics. Much of the fiction examining the advancement of AI technologies builds off of what happens when these laws are pushed to the extreme, or even broken, and AI that was intended to help humanity becomes the enemy. In the most basic sense, much of the culture built in the United States around AI technologies is one of fear.

One of the most famous examples of this fear appears in the *Terminator* franchise where every plotline revolves around defeating Skynet, a self-aware, artificial superintelligence (the farthest point on the Strong AI scale). 1984 saw the release of the first of six movies, and by 2010, the whole franchise composed of movies, television shows, video games, comics, theme park rides, and likely every form of merchandise imaginable had grossed over $3 billion in revenue.[5] Two more movies in the franchise have been released since then. To the United States population, there is something compelling about the idea of an AI, in this case Skynet, being evil. And it's not only the *Terminator* franchise that built a massive fanbase off this idea. *The Matrix* franchise is another multi-billion-dollar United States pop culture staple

---

4. Isaac Asimov, "Runaround" *I, Robot*. Greenwich, CT: Fawcett Publications, 1950.
5. Business Wire, "Pacificor Names Latham & Watkins to Field Terminator Inquiries," *Berkshire Hathaway*, February 17, 2010, https://web.archive.org/web/20170306034914/ http://www.businesswire.com/news/home/20100217005514/en/Pacificor-Names-Latham-Watkins-Field-Terminator-Inquiries.

centered around the story of human society falling to rogue AI. Along with these two franchises come countless one-off movies, television series, and books featuring evil AI systems. The trope is so popular in United States media that lists of favorite "killer AIs" can feature entries from everything from hard-hitting science fiction to children's cartoons.[6]

Not everywhere in the world shares this view of AI. Japan's view of AI technologies is almost completely opposite to the fear of AI seen in United States pop culture. Media in Japan largely portrays robots and Strong AI technologies as friends or in many cases, lovers.[7] This vastly different approach to AI has been attributed to a difference in overall culture, stemming from the different religious framework found in Japan.[8] The history of Buddhism and Shinto in Japan has led society to think of all things, both sentient and non-sentient, as worthy of respect rather than the Judeo-Christian notions of human hierarchy above all except God.[9] Due to this ability to see life in all things, Japanese society was then able to see life in AI and robotics, leading them to quickly view these technologies as the friends and lovers depicted in their media. Even in conversations about the medical AI technologies seen in Japan, the willingness to accept such technology has been directly attributed to the 1950s cartoon, *Astro Boy*.[10]

Unlike the friendliness of AI seen in Japan, the warnings of AI inherent in United States pop culture are not subtle. There is a sense of inevitability in these massive franchises that one day, science will go too far and AI that is meant to be helpful will one day turn on humanity, no matter whether the Three Laws are present in its code or other safety measures are taken. It's no wonder an online scholarly search of the keywords "artificial intelligence" and "too far" within Western publications returns with over 39,000 results.[11] However, these fears have not halted the progress of real-world AI technologies. This development has not always been successful, but each unsuccessful attempt is a step closer to success.

---

6. Andrew Dyce, "Our 10 Favorite Killer A.I.'s in Movies," *Screen Rant*, April 18, 2014. https://screenrant.com/artificial-intelligence-movies-evil-computers/.
7. Cat Ana, "Why the Japanese Find Deep Love with Deep Learning," *Medium* (*Becoming Human: Artificial Intelligence Magazine*, February 12, 2019), https://becominghuman.ai/why-the-japanese-find-deep-love-with-deep-learning-829e1bb629c2.
8. Joi Ito, "Why Westerners Fear Robots and the Japanese Do Not," *Wired* (Conde Nast, July 30, 2018), https://www.wired.com/story/ideas-joi-ito-robot-overlords/
9. Joi Ito, "Why Westerners."
10. Don Lee, "Desperate for Workers, Aging Japan Turns to Robots for Healthcare," *Los Angeles Times*, July 25, 2019, https://www.latimes.com/world-nation/story/2019-07-25/desperate-for-workers-aging-japan-turns-to-robots-for-healthcare.
11. Results from a Google Scholar search on April 11, 2020, excluding patents and citations.

In a "simple" attempt to create an AI that functioned just as well as a human social media presence, Microsoft quickly found their bot was not up to the task. The AI, Tay, was introduced on Twitter in 2016 with her own account, but the experiment was pulled after a mere sixteen hours, which was enough time for Tay to go from a friendly chatbot to using racist slurs.[12] Facial recognition software, even though it's a version of AI many of us use on our current cell phones, has also shown to be less than reliable when implemented on a large scale. For example, China's widescale attempt to ticket jaywalkers in the interest of public safety ended up quickly racking up tickets for models and actors whose faces were advertised on the sides of public transportation.[13] When it is not a face being identified, but rather a single item, some non-specialized identification technology has not had the best outcome either. In one example, a turtle was mistaken for a gun.[14] But for every documented failure such as these, there exists a step toward progress.

In recent years, AI technologies that seem straight out of a science fiction novel and are closer to what would be considered Strong AI have seen great success. Google's AI might have mistaken a turtle for a gun, but there are many specialized item identification apps available that are capable of allowing the average person to identify even rare animal or plant species around them.[15] It's also not only animals in the backyard that have been impacted by AI advancement, with AI-equipped drones being used to halt poaching activities in Africa.[16] Cities have also begun looking to AI for ways to solve existing problems. Los Angeles has turned to AI as a source for a solution to its aging, vulnerable plumbing systems.[17] AI may not be perfect in all aspects

12. James Vincent, "Twitter Taught Microsoft's Friendly AI Chatbot to Be a Racist Asshole in Less Than a Day." *The Verge*. March 24, 2016. https://www.theverge.com/2016/3/24/11297050/tay-microsoft-chatbot-racist.

13. Melanie Ehrenkranz, "Facial Recognition Flags Woman on Bus Ad for 'Jaywalking' in China." *Gizmodo*. November 26, 2018. https://gizmodo.com/facial-recognition-flags-woman-on-bus-ad-for-jaywalking-1830654750.

14. James Vincent, Google's AI Thinks This Turtle Looks like a Gun, Which Is a Problem." *The Verge*. November 2, 2017. https://www.theverge.com/2017/11/2/16597276/google-ai-image-attacks-adversarial-turtle-rifle-3d-printed.

15. Emily Matchar, "AI Plant and Animal Identification Helps Us All Be Citizen Scientists," Smithsonian.com (Smithsonian Institution, June 7, 2017), https://www.smithsonianmag.com/innovation/ai-plant-and-animal-identification-helps-us-all-be-citizen-scientists-180963525/.

16. Builddie, "The Role of Artificial Intelligence in Wildlife Conservation," *Medium*, May 15, 2019, https://medium.com/builddie/the-role-of-artificial-intelligence-in-wildlife-conservation-5dc3af2b4222.

17. Gary Polakovic, "The next Big Effort in AI: Keeping L.A.'s Water Flowing Post-Earthquake," *USC News*, October 4, 2019, https://news.usc.edu/160680/ai-la-water-supply-earthquake-usc-research/.

and further development is still needed to prevent AI from failing as horribly as the bot Tay, but consumer AI technologies have found success. In the medical field, the story of newly developed AI is no different. Some attempts have been more successful than others, but the technology in a large sense has continued to advance. Throughout this progression, the use of AI in a medical setting has raised ethical concerns, even when the utilization of an AI technology has been successful. These concerns have only grown as AI begins to move closer to the side of Strong AI and AI systems begin to overlap in spaces previously reserved for human clinicians only. In this overlap exists the concern that AI will replace a clinician, thereby disrupting the ethics found within the well-established framework of principlism, the most prevalent ethical framework of modern medicine, particularly within the United States.

Beauchamp and Childress' work on principlism details an ethical framework based around how the clinician interacts with the patient. The four principles—nonmaleficence, beneficence, justice, and autonomy—guide how a clinician should interact with, support, or provide for a patient.[18] This relationship between a clinician and a patient is therefore key to the ethical practice of medicine. When the patient-clinician relationship is established, a sense of trustworthiness is created.[19] As said in *The Principles of Biomedical Ethics*, "nothing is more important in healthcare organizations than the maintenance of a culture of trust."[20] Literature discussed later in this paper indicate that worries about the introduction of AI in the medical field revolve around concerns of trust, largely boiling down to fears that a patient would be unable to trust any diagnoses, treatment, or interaction with an AI entity. These concerns have arisen throughout the history of AI in medicine, starting with early research.

In the 1970s, the medical field got its first glimpse at the implementation of AI technologies. MYCIN, an early AI system designed by Stanford School of Medicine researchers, was used to identify certain bacteria such as meningitis and bacteremia and suggest treatment options to prevent severe infection.[21] A full decade before the invention of the internet, MYCIN was able to create a treatment plan with a 65% acceptability rating according to

18. Thomas L. Beauchamp and James F. Childress, *Principles of Biomedical Ethics*. New York: Oxford University Press, 2013.
19. Mark A. Hall et al., "Trust in Physicians and Medical Institutions: What Is It, Can It Be Measured, and Does It Matter?," *The Milbank Quarterly* 79, no. 4 (2001): 613.
20. Beauchamp and Childress, *Principles*, 40.
21. V. L. Yu, "Antimicrobial Selection by a Computer. A Blinded Evaluation by Infectious Diseases Experts," *JAMA: The Journal of the American Medical Association* 242, no. 12 (1979): 1279–282.

the study's parameters. In comparison, five faculty members were asked to create a treatment plan based on the same data and the acceptability ratings assigned to those plans fell between 42.5% and 62.5%. Even with such promising results, the ethics of MYCIN's use were immediately called into question due to an individualized treatment plan being determined by probability modeling rather than an actual physician.[22] In short, how could a machine create an accurate plan if it did not have a relationship with the patient in order to determine what treatment plan would be effective? Although MYCIN was never implemented in a medical setting, these initial questions persisted as AI advanced and began to gain a foothold in medical settings.

The most prevalent attempts to entwine AI with Western medicine can be found in clinical decision support systems (CDSS), specifically diagnostic decision support systems (DDSS.) The intent behind DDSS is to interpret data in order to aid clinicians. Assistance offered through DDSS can, in theory, then help a clinician better diagnose a medical problem by identifying conditions and warning signs of developing conditions in order to flag them for a clinician to view.[23] The field most impacted by DDSS at this point has been radiology, due to the technology's application to medical imaging systems such as MRIs and CAT scans. Traditional methods of examining medical images can result in misdiagnoses, resulting in the need for second opinions which can sometimes complicate the matter further.[24] Additionally, these methods also leave clinicians increasingly exhausted by the end of their shifts, leading to fewer accurate diagnoses as the shift progresses.[25] DDSS that have already been developed and those on the horizon of implementation in the medical field are meant to alleviate some of these issues by providing a real-time second opinion. The DDSS can provide immediate suggestions in these cases, but it is the clinician who makes the final decision on diagnosis and treatment.

Building off the excitement around the idea of DDSS being fully incorporated into the medical field, IBM introduced arguably one of the most

22. David E. Heckerman, and Edward H. Shortliffe, "From Certainty Factors to Belief Networks," *Artificial Intelligence in Medicine* 4, no. 1 (1992): 37.

23. Eta S. Berner and Tonya J. La Lande, "Overview of Clinical Decision Support Systems," in *Clinical Decision Support Systems: Theory and Practice*, ed. Eta S. Berner (Switzerland: Springer International Press, 2016), 3.

24. Christopher Eakins et al., "Second Opinion Interpretations by Specialty Radiologists at a Pediatric Hospital: Rate of Disagreement and Clinical Implications," *American Journal of Roentgenology* 199, no. 4 (2012): pp. 916-920.

25. Elizabeth A. Krupinski et al., "Long Radiology Workdays Reduce Detection and Accommodation Accuracy," *Journal of the American College of Radiology* 7, no. 9 (2010): pp. 698–704

famous examples of AI being used in medical diagnostics—Watson for Oncology. IBM's Watson, a computer capable of understanding natural language and content, was developed far beyond its original purpose in order to introduce the technology to the medical field.[26] Watson was initially designed to compete against human contestants in the television game show, *Jeopardy!*, and ultimately found success in its victory over Ken Jennings, a *Jeopardy!* "greatest of all time," in 2011.[27] After such a public win for AI technologies, IBM shifted the focus of Watson toward medicine, finally releasing Watson for Oncology in 2016.[28] Touted as the next frontier of medicine, Watson was portrayed as an AI system capable of not only assisting in the interpretation of diagnostic imaging, but also capable of supplying actual, effective treatment plans without approval from a clinician. Proponents of AI looked to Watson for Oncology as a way to prove the benefits of introducing more advanced AI into the field of medicine, but still, ethical concerns around a machine making medical decisions were prevalent.[29] As later learned through internal messages from IBM made public in July of 2018, many of these concerns regarding the use of Watson for Oncology were valid.

A STAT report revealed that IBM executives were well aware of the problems found within Watson for Oncology's systems, highlighting that Watson provided "multiple examples of unsafe and incorrect treatment recommendations."[30] Many of these problems were not unknown to IBM employees. Records show that IBM attempted to contact clinicians to notify them of Watson's "very limited" abilities.[31] These attempts were largely unsuccessful and hospital systems continued to operate under the assumption that Watson was providing valid treatment options for patients. After the STAT report was released and Watson's unsafe treatment plans came to light, many hospital systems rushed to issue statements to assuage fears

26. IBM, "Watson Overview," The DeepQA Research Team, July 25, 2016, https://researcher.watson.ibm.com/researcher/view_group.php?id=2099.
27. Eric Brown, "Watson: The *Jeopardy!* Challenge and beyond," 2013 *IEEE 12th International Conference on Cognitive Informatics and Cognitive Computing*, 2013.
28. IBM Newsroom, "Manipal Hospitals Announces National Launch of IBM Watson for Oncology," July 26, 2016, https://www-03.ibm.com/press/in/en/pressrelease/50290.wss.
29. Jennifer Bresnick, "Artificial Intelligence in Healthcare Market to See 40% CAGR Surge," HealthITAnalytics, July 24, 2017, https://healthitanalytics.com/news/artificial-intelligence-in-healthcare-market-to-see-40-cagr-surge.
30. Casey Ross and Ike Swetlitz, "IBM's Watson supercomputer recommended 'unsafe and incorrect' cancer treatments, internal documents show," *STAT*, July 25, 2018.
31. Julie Spitzer, "IBM's Watson recommended 'unsafe and incorrect' cancer treatments, STAT report finds," *Becker's Healthcare*, July 25, 2018.

that AI had gone too far and had replaced the clinician in medical decision making. In a statement reassuring the public that Watson had only been used as a tool, not a decision maker, one hospital spokesperson said, "No technology can replace a doctor and his or her knowledge about their individual patient."[32] The message is clear: the patient-clinician relationship was not weakened through the use of Watson for Oncology because clinicians weren't actually using the AI system to make important decisions; those decisions were entirely the clinicians. However, even after the accuracy of Watson's oncology decisions were called into question, the software is still being implemented in healthcare systems today, including in at least seventy Veterans Affairs Medical Centers (VAMCs) in the United States.[33]

Watson for Oncology's continued use is not the only sign that healthcare systems are still interested in exploring AI's function in the medical field. Yes, AI assisted diagnosis has been implemented—along with assurances that it's still the clinician who is actually making the final call—but companies around the world are developing AI technologies that push further into the medical domain. So far, in fact, that very real concerns have arisen regarding AI replacing clinicians.[34] Currently, there are multiple programs that have been able to successfully complete medical board examinations.

The first country to see an AI pass a medical licensing exam was China in 2017. The AI-equipped robot Xiaoyi, Mandarin for "Little Doctor," made headlines for scoring 456 points of 600 on China's medical licensing exam, a full 96 points above a passing grade.[35] It is important to note that the Chinese exam cannot be passed with rote memorization alone. The exam is structured so that hopeful clinicians must examine cases and determine the appropriate answer based on the information given, therefore showing that they can interpret the information presented to them and make an informed, educated decision.[36] Xiaoyi's first attempt at passing the exam hints at the difficulty of the exam, with the AI only earning a score of

32. Spitzer, "IBM's Watson."

33. Eliza Strickland, "How IBM Watson Overpromised and Underdelivered on AI Health Care," *IEEE Spectrum: Technology, Engineering, and Science News*, April 2, 2019, https://spectrum.ieee.org/biomedical/diagnostics/how-ibm-watson-overpromised-and-underdelivered-on-ai-health-care.

34. Kyle E. Karches, "Against the iDoctor: Why Artificial Intelligence Should Not Replace Physician Judgment," *Theoretical Medicine and Bioethics* 39 (2): 92

35. Ma Si, and Cheng Yu, "Chinese Robot Becomes World's First Machine to Pass Medical Exam," *China Daily*, November 10, 2017, http://www.chinadaily.com.cn/business/tech/2017-11/10/content_34362656.htm.

36. Alice Yan, "How a Robot Passed China's Medical Licensing Exam," *South China Morning Post*, November 20, 2017, accessed April 20, 2019.

slightly above 100. Before the next attempt was made, the research team made Xiaoyi "study" by introducing the robot to numerous textbooks and medical case files.[37] Like all other clinicians who passed the exam during that time, Xiaoyi needed to learn in order to pass the written exam. However, when Xiaoyi demonstrated that the AI was certainly knowledgeable of medical ailments, the research team was quick to announce that Xiaoyi was only able to "make suggestions to doctors, to help them identify problems quicker and avoid some risks."[38] Even though the AI passed a licensing exam, it still needed to be made clear that patients would receive their care from human clinicians, not an AI.

A very different reaction was seen the next time an AI passed a medical board examination. In June of 2018, Babylon Health's AI passed the UK's Membership of the Royal College of General Practitioner's (MRCGP) exam. The MRCGP is the last in a series of exams meant to test medical student's knowledge of the field they are eager to enter. In short, passing the MRCGP means a medical student is finally, after many years of study, ready to practice medicine independently. The average score from 2012 to 2017 was 72%. Babylon's AI scored an 81%.[39] In a statement released after the success of Babylon's AI, Babylon's founder and CEO, Dr. Ali Parsa, did not reassure people that this technology would not replace clinicians or was not able to make medical decisions directly with a patient. In fact, he did the opposite. Pointing out that there are many areas where the ability to see a clinician is extremely limited and the healthcare systems are overloaded, Dr. Parsa claimed the AI's successful completion of the MRCGP "clearly illustrated how AI-augmented health services can reduce the burden on healthcare systems around the world."[40] A shift in the narrative is clear with Babylon AI's success; the future role of AI in medicine may not be as a tool for clinicians to consult, but may very well act as the clinician itself.

Recent changes to the field of medicine have shown that Dr. Parsa's vision for the future use of AI may very well come to pass. Currently, one area of medicine growing exponentially is telemedicine and with that growth comes conversations regarding the changing nature of how medicine is delivered

---

37. Si and Yu, "Chinese Robot."
38. Yan, "How a Robot."
39. Babylon Health, "Babylon AI Achieves Equivalent Accuracy with Human Doctors in Global Healthcare First," *PR Newswire: News Distribution, Targeting and Monitoring,* June 27, 2018.
40. Babylon Health, "Babylon AI Achieves Equivalent Accuracy with Human Doctors."

to patients.[41] In the United States, telehealth options, defined in one study as "videoconferencing, remote monitoring, electronic consults, and wireless communications," were offered to patients through their hospital systems increased from 35% to 76% in the years between 2010 and 2017.[42] One common aspect of telemedicine is the option for virtual appointments like those offered through the Cleveland Clinic, meant to treat basic, frontline illnesses such as the common cold, allergies, and even the flu that do not necessarily require a patient to meet with a clinician face-to-face—the precise kind of appointment Babylon's Dr. Parsa referenced in his statement on the possible applications of Babylon's AI.[43]

People within the United States have begun to grow more comfortable seeking medical advice and treatment through technology. Examples from around the country and the world demonstrate that individuals are not only willing to work with a human via technology but may be willing to see AI technologies as a stand-in for the clinician. One of the most prominent examples in current medical practice is the use of therapy chatbots. These chatbots have been shown to help patients better understand their diagnosis as well as adhere to their treatment plan.[44] Another study showed that patients dealing with post-traumatic stress were more open and able to acknowledge their trauma when disclosing their symptoms to a chatbot than an in-person appointment.[45] It is not as if this particular version of AI in healthcare is ready to replace our current therapy models though.

While participants in studies have been willing to speak to a chatbot and have revealed more than they might initially with an in-person or video call therapy appointment, research has shown that there may be some caveats. In particular, some studies have indicated that some individuals are willing to disclose more information to a chatbot only once they know a human clinician will go back to read over the transcript at a later time.[46] That being

---

41. Tommaso Iannitti et al., "Narrative Review of Telemedicine Consultation in Medical Practice," *Patient Preference and Adherence*, 2015, 65.
42. American Hospital Association, "Fact Sheet: Telehealth," February 2019.
43. "Cleveland Clinic Express Care® Online," Cleveland Clinic, 2019.
44. Aditya Vaidyam and John Torous. "Chatbots: What Are They and Why Care?" *Psychiatric Times*, June 27, 2019. https://www.psychiatrictimes.com/telepsychiatry/chatbots-what-are-they-and-why-care.
45. Myrthe L. Tielman et al., "A Therapy System for Post-Traumatic Stress Disorder Using a Virtual Agent and Virtual Storytelling to Reconstruct Traumatic Memories," *Journal of Medical Systems* 41, no. 8 (2017): 125.
46. Timothy W. Bickmore et al., "Response to a Relational Agent by Hospital Patients with Depressive Symptoms," *Interacting with Computers* 22, no. 4 (2010): 289.

said, even though these participants found comfort in knowing any final psychological diagnoses or therapeutic feedback would come from a human clinician, they were still willing to work with an AI during the beginning of the treatment process for that session. And considering the commercial success of therapy apps and the fact that the American Psychiatric Association has begun tracking and rating the potential effectiveness of these apps, often containing a chatbot component, there is little reason to think people will not utilize this technology more in the future.[47]

The idea of a virtual therapist poses a different dynamic than the traditional model, even if there is a human clinician at the end of the process. With this new model, the clinician-patient relationship begins to look different from the face-to-face, human-to-human interactions described by Beauchamp and Childress. Although participants still wanted to be sure that the end decider was human, the initial relationship-building was not with a human, but rather an AI. This marks a divergence from the attitudes seen toward DDSS like Watson for Oncology that function behind the scenes. Those AI systems are designed to be used as tools behind the scenes and in conjunction with a clinician's expertise. A virtual chatbot designed for therapy interacts with the human first and later relays information gathered from a human to another human. These chatbot AIs are not looking at images, they are working with dialogue and building a relationship with a client. The relationship may not look directly like the clinician-patient relationship modern medicine has developed, but in these circumstances, AI is undeniably becoming entwined in the relationship between a patient and a clinician. And while the mentioned chatbots obviously cannot replace an in-person interaction with a clinician, other technologies being developed in the world are beginning to push against that boundary as well.

In Japan where AI is already seen in a favorable light, AI technologies helping patients in a direct manner have gone one step further than online therapists. Japan has started implementing AI-equipped care robots that are capable of doling out the correct dosage of medications and seeing to the basic needs of their aging population in ways as simple as adjusting the temperature in their rooms.[48] The demand has grown so great for robotics

47. Jessica Truschel, "Top 25 Mental Health Apps for 2020: An Alternative to Therapy?," Psycom.net– Mental Health Treatment Resource Since 1986, March 19, 2020, https://www.psycom.net/25-best-mental-health-apps.

48. Naomi Tajitsu, "Japanese Automakers Look to Robots to Aid the Elderly," *Scientific American*. April 12, 2017, https://www.scientificamerican.com/article/japanese-automakers-look-to-robots-to-aid-the-elderly.

within the geriatric care field that many automakers have turned away from designing autonomous vehicles and are instead providing technologies such as beds that transform into wheelchairs or cybernetic legs that allow the care workers to lift heavy patients on their own.[49] In more direct, personal ways, AI-equipped humanoid robots such as SoftBank Robotics' Pepper have also been developed to sing to elderly patients and also answer basic questions such as "where is the bathroom?"[50] Even Japanese-designed companion animals such as the robotic seal, Paro, have been explicitly created to react to human interaction and provide the means for elderly patients to build a relationship with a non-living entity.[51]

Technologies such as Paro and Pepper are intentionally designed to capitalize on the distinct cultural ability for Japanese patients to connect with AI and have seen great success because of this. Considering this previously discussed ability for Japanese individuals to view AI in a positive light, it no surprise they are on the forefront of adopting AI in a healthcare setting. In these examples, the technology was implemented to meet the needs of Japan's aging population by addressing the lack of available care workers. By utilizing the AI technology in that environment, Japanese humanoid AI robots meet the first requirement to implement AI in a healthcare setting ethically. The second requirement of ensuring the ability to maintain the patient-clinician relationship is partially met, as the patients have demonstrated a clear ability to connect with these technologies, but not in the manner of patient and decision-making clinician. While the humanoid AI in Japan does not fully reach to the levels of future technology that could be implemented within a healthcare setting, these current technologies are certainly a step in that direction.

Overall, the United States might not be ready for the large-scale implementation of AI-equipped humanoid robotics like those seen in Japan. Rather, AI technology more realistically adaptable to United States healthcare systems would be something more akin to Babylon's AI where the AI would act as a frontline clinician. As a frontline clinician, AI would quickly diagnose basic ailments such as colds and flu and would refer to a human clinician or specialist when necessary. AI of that caliber could be implemented in the United States while adhering with the two ethical requirements of meeting a documented need and maintaining the patient-clinician relationship.

---

49. Don Lee, "Desperate for Workers."
50. Don Lee, "Desperate for Workers."
51. Amy Harmon, "A Soft Spot for Circuitry," *The New York Times.* July 5, 2010, https://www.nytimes.com/2010/07/05/science/05robot.html?_r=2&pagewanted=1.

At least regarding concerns related to an aging population, the United States healthcare system is seeing the same needs as those addressed with AI in Japan. There are growing worries in the United States that there is not enough support available to elderly patients and this concern was addressed in a March 2019 report released by the Trump Administration.[52] The report, *Emerging Technologies to Support an Aging Population,* clearly indicates the current healthcare model is simply not working and emerging technologies should be implemented in order to ease the burden placed on current health providers. By implementing technology, the United States would be less reliant on home healthcare aids which is a growing field due to the sheer numbers of people needing care, but concerns about low pay and the physical demands of the job are likely to continue contributing to a dearth of home healthcare aides within the workforce.[53] The lack of available care of the United States' population is certainly not the only environment where documented shortfalls in current care may be or have already been addressed with technology.

Rural populations pose a particular challenge for the modern model of healthcare. With more centralized hospital systems focused around the nation's largest cities, clinicians have been pulled further away from the ideal of the small-town doctor able to make house calls. The challenges brought forth by patients in remote areas has led to calls for telemedicine options to be more readily available.[54] By implementing the ability for patients to see a doctor virtually, patients do not have to drive to the nearest health facility, find transportation when a car is not readily available, or rely on a clinician to travel to them. Babylon Health has explicitly targeted opportunities to assist these remote populations. After passing the UK medical licensing exam, Babylon's AI was rolled out for remote populations in Africa, allowing a system where there are too few clinicians to see a greater number of patients and more importantly, spend more time with patients who need additional care.[55] Babylon has grown since then, with the London-based

---

52. Mark Mather, Paola Scommegna, and Lillian Kilduff, "Fact Sheet: Aging in the United States," Population Reference Bureau, July 15, 2019, https://www.prb.org/aging-unitedstates-fact-sheet/.

53. U.S. Bureau of Labor Statistics, "Home Health Aides and Personal Care Aides: Occupational Outlook Handbook," September 4, 2019. https://www.bls.gov/ooh/healthcare/home-health-aides-and-personal-care-aides.htm.

54. Ahmed Hosney and Hugo J. W. L. Aerts, "Artificial Intelligence for Global Health." American Association for the Advancement of Science, November 22, 2019, https://science.sciencemag.org/content/366/6468/955.full.

55. Babylon Health, "Babylon AI Achieves Equivalent Accuracy with Human Doctors."

company developing an iOS and Android app intended to get that same frontline healthcare into the hands of anyone in the United States with a smartphone. The idea behind the technology is a simple one—in a system where access to healthcare is a challenge, find a way to increase access.

If AI as a frontline clinician can interact with a patient and diagnose common illnesses and ailments such as allergies, the common cold, or even the flu, then human patient-clinician interaction can, in theory, be reserved for more complicated matters. Since the clinician would not need to reserve time in order to see patients who could be diagnosed quickly and easily with the use of AI, the clinician would then be able to have a longer, more in-depth conversation with patients in need of more specific care. Not only would this maintain a patient-clinician relationship between a human and a frontline AI medical decision-maker, but also increase the patient-clinician relationship between the human patient and the human clinician. However, many have been quick to point out a problem in a model where AI is the end decision maker for medical diagnosis, even for simple matters. Known as the black box problem, the worry is that should a patient's diagnosis come from an AI, even if the end decision seems to make sense, there is no way for a human to understand *why* that diagnosis was made.[56]

The black box nature of AI may be seen as frustrating due to the inability to fully grasp why an AI made the decision it did, but this frustration is likely born from past medical practices regarding patient-clinician relationships. The black box problem poses a very similar ethical issue as was seen with the prevalence of paternalistic approaches to medicine. The AI makes a decision, and the patient would be expected to accept that decision without question. As medicine progressed, an increased desire for autonomy in medical decision making was seen in order for patients in the Western healthcare environment to have more control over their own medical care.[57] However, future technologies may not have this same problem as AI improves. The AI may make the decision, but by identifying the black box problem now, it well within the realm of possibility that researchers will design future AI technologies to have the ability to explain why certain conclusions were reached based on given data. Such progress would be a remarkable move from Weak AI to Strong AI and to reexamine the previous examples of

---

56. Robin C. Feldman, Ehrik Aldana, and Kara Stein. 2019. "Artificial Intelligence in the Health Care Space: How can we trust what we cannot know," *Stanford Law & Policy Review* 30 (2): 406.
57. Beauchamp and Childress, *Principles*, 220.

diagnostic systems and AI systems passing medical licensing exams, steps toward this progress are already happening.

Without devolving into a full argument of the potential for paternalism within AI versus remaining paternalistic habits of human clinicians who aim for beneficence, there is one additional point suggesting that the black box should not be considered a significant flaw of AI technologies. Quite simply, if an AI is not able to fully explain to a patient why a decision was reached, it is not wholly different from a specialist attempting to fully explain their reasoning to a patient with no medical knowledge. Miscommunications and misunderstandings between clinicians and their patients are well documented in literature, indicating that even though a clinician theoretically possess the means to explain their decision, they do not always do so accurately.[58] All this indicates, however, is that no matter whether it's a human clinician or a future AI delivering a diagnosis directly to a patient, steps must be taken in order prevent miscommunication and maintain trust between the patient and their care provider. With developing AI systems, researchers should strive to mitigate the black box problem, but it's current existence within AI does not itself indicate without a doubt that the technology is unethical.

Even in a future where the black box problem is overcome or we as a society fully trust the AI's decision without explanation, other realistic problems of the use of AI still remain. One of the most prominent concerns of individuals relying on AI rather than their own expertise is the possibility that a person will ignore their own intelligence and rely on the technology, even when it is clearly wrong. An example of this phenomenon already seen with AI is that of the many people who have followed their GPS directions straight into a body of water.[59] Those people ignored their own sense of direction, ignored all signs indicating the paths they were driving down were not meant for them, and followed the instructions of their GPS, ultimately finding themselves submerged. While no one was injured in these situations and the end result is a damaged car, a bit of embarrassment, and a decent headline for the local newspaper the next day, not all instances of reliance on faulty technology are as innocent. To once again mention Watson for Oncology, it ultimately became clear that

---

58. Dennis Rosen. *Vital Conversations: Improving Communication Between Doctors and Patients.* New York: Columbia University Press, 2014, 161–162.
59. Malone Kircher. "Yet Another Person Listens to GPS App and Drives Car into Lake." *Intelligencer*, January 24, 2018. https://nymag.com/intelligencer/2018/01/waze-app-directs-driver-to-drive-car-into-lake-champlain.html.

the proposed treatment plans would not be effective for patients and may have done more harm than good. Had clinicians only listened to the AI's suggestions rather than used their own medical training to recognize when something didn't make sense regarding the patient's treatment, it very well could have led to a patient's death. A death caused directly by inaccurate information given by an AI and a clinician's trust that the AI "knew better."

The black box problem and the potential for a clinician to ignore their own training and completely defer to an AI implemented in a health system are certainly issues to address as AI inevitably becomes further entwined in medical decision making. However, these concerns should not prevent the application of future technologies in healthcare systems. Acknowledging that based on the current trends of AI technologies around the globe and in the United States, it is imperative to discuss the ethical applications of near-future technologies. As stated, a logical next step of AI in healthcare is that of AI as a frontline clinician. The key to ethically implementing such AI systems within a medical setting is twofold: the AI must fill a need within the healthcare setting and the patient must be able to connect with the AI in order to preserve the patient-clinician relationship. There may be specific doctor's offices or a certain branch of a hospital system that might me some facets of this criteria, but there is one United States healthcare system as a whole that would provide the groundwork for the ethical application of frontline AI clinicians—the Veterans Health Administration (VHA).

To address the first need in the ethical use of AI as a frontline clinician, the VHA has a well-documented history of long wait times, inadequate care, and an overall reputation of not meeting the needs of its patients. Even the process of receiving benefits through the VHA can be a nightmare for some service members of the United States Armed Forces. In particularly atrocious examples of the VHA's mishandling of disability claims, one man who had received documented injuries during his time in the Coast Guard spent thirty-four years appealing the Department of Veterans Affairs for disability benefits.[60] Another veteran with diabetes had to fight for care, ultimately losing a foot and by the time her claim was approved, her other foot had been amputated as well.[61] Even when a veteran is granted approval to seek care or receive payment, problems remain.

---

60. Dave Philipps, "Veterans Claiming Disability Pay Face Wall of Denials and Delays," *The New York Times*, November 13, 2017, https://www.nytimes.com/2017/11/13/us/veterans-affairs-department-benefits-delays.html.
61. Dave Phillips, "Veterans Claiming Disability Pay."

The VHA has a history of veterans unable to schedule timely appointments, even for life-threatening illnesses.[62] This concern made headlines around the United States when CNN released a report on the Veterans' Affairs healthcare system in Phoenix, AZ, where veterans died due to their inability to be seen by a clinician. CNN exposed that these deaths were the result of a "secret list" created by VHA managers to hide the fact that around 1,500 patients were forced to wait months to see a doctor, ultimately killing at least forty veterans due to lack of care.[63] The VHA has taken steps to identify areas where wait times exceed their requirement that patients be seen in a timely manner, but difficulties arise in trying to define what constitutes a long wait time for patients as well as contending with a system that will schedule an appointment for a veteran, but ultimately reschedule the appointment many times.[64] Progress has been made since the scandal in Phoenix, but wait times are still a concern for the VHA even with the steps taken over the last several years to improve scheduling systems and increase oversight.[65] While the actual act of scheduling (and often rescheduling) has been cited as a reason for long wait times, another issue is a lack of care providers.

Estimates have suggested that by 2025, there will be a nationwide clinician shortage in the United States, particularly affecting rural hospital systems and those that are unable to provide competitive salaries.[66] Unfortunately, the VHA often falls into both of those categories causing increased concerns for under supported VAMCs. Potential problems caused by a future clinician shortage have already been seen in the VHA. From the years 2011 to 2015, the number of clinicians leaving the VHA increased

62. *Waiting for Care: Examining Patient Wait Times at VA Committee on Veterans' Affairs Committee on Veterans' Affairs*, 2013, Statement of Chairman Mike Coffman, Subcommittee on Oversight and Investigations of Veterans' Affairs. http://search.ebscohost.com/login.aspx?direct=true&AuthType=ip,shib&db=cat07006a&AN=cwru.b4081068&site=eds-live.
63. Scott Bronstein and Drew Griffin, "A Fatal Wait: Veterans Languish and Die on a VA Hospital's Secret List," *CNN* (Cable News Network, April 24, 2014), https://www.cnn.com/2014/04/23/health/veterans-dying-health-care-delays/index.html.
64. Brendan McGarry, "VA Audit Confirms Veterans' Wait Times Complaints," Military.com, 2014, https://www.military.com/daily-news/2014/06/10/va-audit-confirms-veterans-wait-times-complaints.html.
65. Patricia Kime, "5 Years After Nationwide Scandal, VA Still Struggles to Track Wait Times," Military.com, July 26, 2019, https://www.military.com/daily-news/2019/07/26/5-years-after-nationwide-scandal-va-still-struggles-track-wait-times.html
66. Department of Health and Human Services, Health Resources and Services Administration, Designated Health Professional Shortage Areas Statistic, HRSA Data Warehouse, 2017.

every fiscal year due to retirements and voluntary resignations.[67] A 2018 report from the United States Government Accountability Office (GAO) clearly demonstrated that the VHA struggles to recruit and retain full-time VHA clinicians and while steps have been taken to improve retention, many VAMCs rely on part-time contracted clinicians, those who volunteer their time, or clinicians in training who ultimately leave.[68] Understandably, the VHA has identified hiring new clinicians as a top priority, but the GAO discovered in 2019 that attempts to increase clinician staffing resulted in more clinicians, yes, but many of them lacked necessary credentialing.[69] In one particularly egregious example given in the report, a clinician who had previously had her license revoked for patient neglect was hired by the VHA. All of these reports of patient wait times, clinician availability, and clinician hiring paint a clear picture—the VHA needs help.

While not all of the challenges faced by the VHA can be resolved by AI, the implementation of AI as a frontline clinician would address many of these established concerns, meeting the first of the two requirements to implement AI as a frontline clinician ethically. Utilizing AI in such a manner would not be the first time AI has been presented as a solution to VHA problems. A 2008 hearing before the Committee on Veterans' Affairs presented a proposal to use AI to increase the VHA's claims processing system.[70] From the previous discussion on processing claims and the Phoenix VHA scandal, the proposals put forth in this hearing did not result in much improvement. However, in 2021, a new software system is scheduled to be implemented throughout the VHA with the intent to vastly improve on current scheduling processes and wait times.[71] It will, of course, take time to see whether adopting AI in the manner of scheduling software will see a reduction in complaints filed related to issues with patients being able to see a clinician in a timely manner. Even if the system makes it easier to track appointment scheduling and create appointments to begin with, the problem of the lack

---

67. *Steps Taken to Improve Physician Staffing, Recruitment, and Retention, but Challenges Remain.* Statement by Director of Health Care, Debra Draper Before the Subcommittee on Health, Committee on Veterans' Affairs, House of Representatives Veterans Health, 2018.
68. *Steps Taken to Improve Physician Staffing.*
69. Kathy Larin, "Veterans health administration: Greater focus on credentialing needed to prevent disqualified providers from delivering patient care," *Nova Science Publishers, Inc.* 2019: 205.
70. *The Use of Artificial Intelligence to Improve the U.S. Department of Veterans Affairs' Claims Processing System,* 2008. Hearing before the Subcommittee on Disability Assistance and Memorial Affairs of the Committee on Veterans' Affairs U.S. House of Representatives
71. Patricia Kime, "5 Years After Nationwide Scandal."

of qualified clinicians will still remain and must be addressed. The current use of Watson for Oncology in more than seventy VAMCs is intended to support clinicians but future implementation of AI as a frontline clinician would directly assist with the overall need for manpower. By using AI as a frontline clinician, VHA patients would be able to schedule immediately with an AI for basic care or to get a referral, freeing up existing clinicians to address the concerns of veterans who need more focused care.

Acknowledging that the use of AI as a frontline clinician would address many of the documented needs of the VHA, the second requirement of the ethical use of such technology still remains. In order to be used ethically, members of the United States Armed Forces must be able to maintain the patient-clinician relationship with an AI as a frontline clinician. Fortunately, during their time of service, many service members have demonstrated an ability to form personal connections with cutting-edge technologies. This is particularly evident with explosive ordinance disposal (EOD) units and their use of bomb-disposal robots that first began in 1972.[72] In the years since these robots were implemented in the field, EOD units have shown a remarkable ability to form emotional bonds with the robot to the point where units will create names for the robot and treat it like a pet.[73] Some units have developed strong enough relationships with their robots that when the robot suffers irreparable damage, the unit will exhibit genuine grief and hold a funeral for their "fellow soldier."[74] Examples from EOD units and their fallen robots may show that soldiers are able to form relationships with non-human entities. Veterans with PTSD, too, have shown a willingness to disclose more information to an AI chatbot than they would in a typical setting.[75] This direct relationship with AI is likely to grow given the military's demonstrated willingness to turn to advancing technology to meet the needs of servicemembers.

Throughout history, military research has been at the forefront of medical advancement. While the root cause for the need to develop such technology

72. Military.com, "The Very First Bomb Disposal Robot," January 15, 2014, https://www.military.com/video/ammunition-and-explosives/explosive-ordnance-disposal/the-first-bomb-disposal-robot/3059244734001.
73. Doree Armstrong, "Emotional Attachment to Robots Could Affect Outcome on Battlefield," Office of Minority Affairs Diversity, September 13, 2013, https://www.washington.edu/news/2013/09/17/emotional-attachment-to-robots-could-affect-outcome-on-battlefield/.
74. Megan Garber, "Funerals for Fallen Robots," *The Atlantic*. September 20, 2013. https://www.theatlantic.com/technology/archive/2013/09/funerals-for-fallen-robots/279861/.
75. Myrthe L. Tielman et al., "A Therapy System for Post-Traumatic Stress Disorder."

is often tragic, the military has always provided an environment in which prosthetic limbs have seen great advancement and methods for salvaging limbs and increasing their functionality has improved.[76] Even things as seemingly basic as the tourniquet or the mass production of antibiotics originated in a military context.[77] These advances went from a military context to entering all healthcare systems and future medical developments can be expected to do the same.

Current declassified research from the Defense Advanced Research Projects Agency (DARPA) indicates an interest in implementing medical AI technologies in the U.S. Armed Forces. One of DARPA's programs, Warfighter Analytics using Smartphones for Health (WASH), aims to use the technology built into a smartphone in order to track the health and overall readiness of a solider, down to identifying minor changes in a soldier's gait, muscle tension, and perspiration level.[78] Another project announced in 2019, Bioelectronics for Tissue Regeneration (BETR), aims to use AI in combination with sensors to track the body's response to biochemical or biophysical stimulations to tissue in order to provide data to actuators that will be able to heal wounds.[79] As military technology advances and AI becomes more integrated in interactions within the military, examples of servicemembers connecting with technology during their time of service will only grow. And in addition to interactions with AI that occur during their time of service, members of the U.S. Armed Forces will also have access to AI technology developed for mass consumers as well.

These interactions with AI then create the foundation on which service members seeking treatment through the VHA can receive treatment in a timely manner and still maintain the patient-clinician relationship with AI acting as the frontline clinician. Understandably, not all service members will have the same level of interaction with AI as others, particularly of elderly patients who did not encounter AI during their time of service. In order to best adhere to an ethical use of AI as a frontline clinician,

76. Melissa Block, "Orthotic Brace Takes Soldiers from Limping to Leaping," *NPR*, March 31, 2014, https://www.npr.org/sections/health-shots/2014/03/31/295328707/orthotic-brace-takes-soldiers-from-limping-to-leaping.

77. Leah Samuel, "6 Battlefield Medical Innovations That Moved to Mainstream Medicine," *STAT*, November 10, 2017, https://www.statnews.com/2017/11/10/medical-innovations-war/.

78. Jonathan M. Smith, "Warfighter Analytics Using Smartphones for Health (WASH)." https://www.darpa.mil/program/warfighter-analytics-using-smartphones-for-health.

79. Dr. Paul Sheehan, "Bioelectronics for Tissue Regeneration (BETR)." https://www.darpa.mil/program/bioelectronics-for-tissue-regeneration.

servicemembers seeking treatment at a VAMC should be given the choice to interact first with an AI or to wait until a human clinician is available. To do otherwise, to ask that an individual who would not be willing to speak to a chatbot or have an AI assist them in diagnosing a cold or flu do so despite their comfort, would harm the patient–clinician relationship and make the implementation of the technology unethical. But given the nature of humanity's progressing relationship with AI overall, and the indications of future application within the U.S. Armed Forces, the coming years will likely see an increase in patients willing to first interact with an AI. As previously discussed in relation to patients with PTSD and their interactions with a chatbot and the overall success of telehealth appointments that are readily available, it may be that patients would rather speak to an AI if it meant they could receive care in that moment.

At the heart of AI's implementation in medicine is a desire to provide better, more accurate, more accessible care. In many ways, proposing the application of AI as a frontline clinician in a United States healthcare system poses a greater challenge due to an ingrained societal mistrust of AI. Ethical concerns rooted in this mistrust have not been able to prevent technological advancement, however and it is now imperative to shift the conversation from "should AI be allowed" to "how should AI be implemented?" To ensure the ethical use of future technologies in a healthcare system, two requirements must be met. The technology must meet a documented need and the implementation of the technology must not damage the potential for the development of the patient–clinician relationship.

The Veterans Health Administration's documented inability to fully care for patients to the established standard could be addressed through the use of AI as a frontline clinician. Not only that, but many members of the U.S. Armed forces who seek care at VAMCs in the future will have interacted with, and developed a unique relationship with, AI technologies during their time of service. These interactions would make them capable of maintaining trust in a medical decision when AI is the clinician, preserving the patient–clinician relationship. AI may not yet fully able to act as a frontline clinician, but it is imperative to identify now how to ethically implement AI in the future. While future AI technologies will undoubtedly improve healthcare overall, the Veterans Health Administration stands to benefit greatly from this technology and provides an environment in which AI's implementation can adhere to principles at the foundation of Western medical ethics.

References

American Hospital Association. "Fact Sheet: Telehealth." February 2019. https://www.aha.org/system/files/2019-02/fact-sheet-telehealth-2-4-19.pdf.

Ana, Cat. "Why the Japanese Find Deep Love with Deep Learning." *Medium. Becoming Human: Artificial Intelligence Magazine*, February 12, 2019. https://becominghuman.ai/why-the-japanese-find-deep-love-with-deep-learning-829e1bb629c2.

Armstrong, Doree. "Emotional Attachment to Robots Could Affect Outcome on Battlefield." Office of Minority Affairs Diversity. September 13, 2013. https://www.washington.edu/news/2013/09/17/emotional-attachment-to-robots-could-affect-outcome-on-battlefield/.

Asimov, Isaac. "Runaround" *I, Robot*. Greenwich, CT: Fawcett Publications, 1950.

Bickmore, Timothy W., Suzanne E. Mitchell, Brian W. Jack, Michael K. Paasche-Orlow, Laura M. Pfeifer, and Julie O'Donnell. "Response to a Relational Agent by Hospital Patients with Depressive Symptoms." *Interacting with Computers* 22, no. 4 (2010): 289–98.

Block, Melissa. "Orthotic Brace Takes Soldiers from Limping to Leaping." *NPR*, March 31, 2014. https://www.npr.org/sections/health-shots/2014/03/31/295328707/orthotic-brace-takes-soldiers-from-limping-to-leaping.

Bronstein, Scott, and Drew Griffin. "A Fatal Wait: Veterans Languish and Die on a VA Hospital's Secret List." *CNN*. Cable News Network, April 24, 2014. https://www.cnn.com/2014/04/23/health/veterans-dying-health-care-delays/index.html.

Builddie. "The Role of Artificial Intelligence in Wildlife Conservation." *Medium*. May 15, 2019. https://medium.com/builddie/the-role-of-artificial-intelligence-in-wildlife-conservation-5dc3af2b4222.

Business Wire. "Pacificor Names Latham & Watkins to Field Terminator Inquiries." Berkshire Hathaway. February 17, 2010. http://www.businesswire.com/news/home/20100217005514/en/Pacificor-Names-Latham-Watkins-Field-Terminator-Inquiries.

Eakins, Christopher, Wendy D. Ellis, Sumit Pruthi, David P. Johnson, Marta Hernanz-Schulman, Chang Yu, and J. Herman Kan. "Second Opinion Interpretations by Specialty Radiologists at a Pediatric Hospital: Rate of Disagreement and Clinical Implications." *American Journal of Roentgenology* 199, no. 4 (2012): 916–20.

Babylon Health, "Babylon AI Achieves Equivalent Accuracy with Human Doctors in Global Healthcare First." PR Newswire: News Distribution, Targeting and Monitoring. June 27, 2018. https://www.prnewswire.com/news-releases/babylon-ai-achieves-equivalent-accuracy-with-human-doctors-in-global-health-care-first-686718631.html.

Beauchamp, Thomas L., and James F. Childress. *Principles of Biomedical Ethics*. New York: Oxford University Press, 2013

Berner, Eta S. and Tonya J. La Lande, "Overview of Clinical Decision Support Systems," in *Clinical Decision Support Systems: Theory and Practice,* ed. Eta S. Berner. Switzerland: Springer International Press, 2016.

Bresnick, Jennifer. "Artificial Intelligence in Healthcare Market to See 40% CAGR Surge." HealthITAnalytics, July 24, 2017. https://healthitanalytics.com/news/artificial-intelligence-in-healthcare-market-to-see-40-cagr-surge.

Brown, Eric. "Watson: The *Jeopardy!* Challenge and beyond." 2013 IEEE 12th International Conference on Cognitive Informatics and Cognitive Computing, 2013.

Brynjolfsson, Erik, and Andrew McAfee. The Second Machine Age: Work, Progress, and Prosperity in a Time of Brilliant Technologies. Vancouver, BC: Langara College, 2018.

"Cleveland Clinic Express Care® Online." Cleveland Clinic. Accessed April 29, 2019. https://my.clevelandclinic.org/online-services/express-care-online.

Dyce, Andrew. "Our 10 Favorite Killer A.I.'s in Movies." Screen Rant, April 18, 2014. https://screenrant.com/artificial-intelligence-movies-evil-computers/.

Ehrenkranz, Melanie. "Facial Recognition Flags Woman on Bus Ad for 'Jaywalking' in China." Gizmodo. November 26, 2018. https://gizmodo.com/facial-recognition-flags-woman-on-bus-ad-for-jaywalking-1830654750.

Feldman, Robin C., Ehrik Aldana, and Kara Stein. 2019. "Artificial Intelligence in the Health Care Space: How can we trust what we cannot know." *Stanford Law & Policy Review* 30 (2): 399–419.

Garber, Megan. "Funerals for Fallen Robots." *The Atlantic.* September 20, 2013. https://www.theatlantic.com/technology/archive/2013/09/funerals-for-fallen-robots/279861/.

Hall, Mark A., Elizabeth Dugan, Beiyao Zheng, and Aneil K. Mishra. "Trust in Physicians and Medical Institutions: What Is It, Can It Be Measured, and Does It Matter?" *The Milbank Quarterly* 79, no. 4 (2001): 613–39.

Harmon, Amy. "A Soft Spot for Circuitry." *The New York Times.* July 5, 2010. https://www.nytimes.com/2010/07/05/science/05robot.html?_r=2&pagewanted=1..

Hosny, Ahmed, and Hugo J. W. L. Aerts. "Artificial Intelligence for Global Health." *American Association for the Advancement of Science,* November 22, 2019. https://science.sciencemag.org/content/366/6468/955.full.

Heckerman, David E., and Edward H. Shortliffe. "From Certainty Factors to Belief Networks." *Artificial Intelligence in Medicine* 4, no. 1 (1992): 35–52.

Iannitti, Tommaso, Alessandro Di Cerbo, Julio Cesar Morales-Medina, and Beniamino Palmieri. "Narrative Review of Telemedicine Consultation in Medical Practice." Patient Preference and Adherence, 2015, 65.

IBM. "Watson Overview." The DeepQA Research Team, July 25, 2016. https://researcher.watson.ibm.com/researcher/view_group.php?id=2099.

IBM Newsroom. "Manipal Hospitals Announces National Launch of IBM Watson for Oncology." IBM, July 26, 2016. https://www-03.ibm.com/press/in/en/pressrelease/50290.wss.

Ito, Joi. "Why Westerners Fear Robots and the Japanese Do Not." Wired. Conde Nast, July 30, 2018. https://www.wired.com/story/ideas-joi-ito-robot-overlords/.

Karches, Kyle E. 2018. "Against the IDoctor: Why Artificial Intelligence Should Not Replace Physician Judgment." *Theoretical Medicine and Bioethics* 39 (2): 91–110.

Kircher, Malone. "Yet Another Person Listens to GPS App and Drives Car Into Lake." *Intelligencer,* January 24, 2018. https://nymag.com/intelligencer/2018/01/waze-app-directs-driver-to-drive-car-into-lake-champlain.html.

Kime, Patricia. "5 Years After Nationwide Scandal, VA Still Struggles to Track Wait Times." Military.com, July 26, 2019. https://www.military.com/daily-news/2019/07/26/5-years-after-nationwide-scandal-va-still-struggles-track-wait-times.html.

Krupinski, Elizabeth A., Kevin S. Berbaum, Robert T. Caldwell, Kevin M. Schartz, and John Kim. "Long Radiology Workdays Reduce Detection and Accommodation Accuracy." *Journal of the American College of Radiology* 7, no. 9 (2010): 698–704.

Larin, Kathy. "Veterans health administration: Greater focus on credentialing needed to prevent disqualified providers from delivering patient care." Nova Science Publishers, Inc. 2019: 205-284.

Lee, Don. "Desperate for Workers, Aging Japan Turns to Robots for Healthcare." *Los Angeles Times.* July 25, 2019. https://www.latimes.com/world-nation/story/2019-07-25/desperate-for-workers-aging-japan-turns-to-robots-for-healthcare.

Matchar, Emily. "AI Plant and Animal Identification Helps Us All Be Citizen Scientists." Smithsonian.com. Smithsonian Institution, June 7, 2017. https://www.smithsonianmag.com/innovation/ai-plant-and-animal-identification-helps-us-all-be-citizen-scientists-180963525/.

Mather, Mark, Paola Scommegna, and Lillian Kilduff. "Fact Sheet: Aging in the United States." Population Reference Bureau, July 15, 2019. https://www.prb.org/aging-unitedstates-fact-sheet/

McGarry, Brendan. "VA Audit Confirms Veterans' Wait Times Complaints." Military.com, 2014. https://www.military.com/daily-news/2014/06/10/va-audit-confirms-veterans-wait-times-complaints.html.

Military.com. "The Very First Bomb Disposal Robot." January 15, 2014. https://www.military.com/video/ammunition-and-explosives/explosive-ordnance-disposal/the-first-bomb-disposal-robot/3059244734001.

National Science and Technology Council. "Emerging Technologies to Support an Aging Population." March 2019. https://www.whitehouse.gov/wp-content/uploads/2019/03/Emerging-Tech-to-Support-Aging-2019.pdf.

Oxford English Dictionary Online. "Artificial Intelligence." November 2019. Oxford: Oxford University Press. https://www.oed.com/view/Entry/271625?redirectedFrom=artificial+intelligence#eid.

Philipps, Dave. "Veterans Claiming Disability Pay Face Wall of Denials and Delays." *The New York Times.* November 13, 2017. https://www.nytimes.com/2017/11/13/us/veterans-affairs-department-benefits-delays.html.

Polakovic, Gary. "The next Big Effort in AI: Keeping L.A.'s Water Flowing Post-Earthquake." USC News, October 4, 2019. https://news.usc.edu/160680/ai-la-water-supply-earthquake-usc-research/.

Ross, Casey, and Ike Swetlitz. "IBM's Watson supercomputer recommended 'unsafe and incorrect' cancer treatments, internal documents show." *STAT,* July 25, 2018. https://www.statnews.com/2018/07/25/ibm-watson-recommended-unsafe-incorrect-treatments/.

Rosen, Dennis. *Vital Conversations: Improving Communication Between Doctors and Patients.* New York: Columbia University Press, 2014.

Russell, Stuart J., and Peter Norvig. *Artificial Intelligence a Modern Approach*. Boston: Pearson, 2016.

Samuel, Leah. "6 Battlefield Medical Innovations That Moved to Mainstream Medicine." STAT, November 10, 2017. https://www.statnews.com/2017/11/10/medical-innovations-war/.

Si, Ma, and Cheng Yu. "Chinese Robot Becomes World's First Machine to Pass Medical Exam." November 10, 2017. http://www.chinadaily.com.cn/bizchina/tech/2017-11/10/content_34362656.htm.

Sheehan, Dr. Paul. "Bioelectronics for Tissue Regeneration (BETR)." https://www.darpa.mil/program/bioelectronics-for-tissue-regeneration..

Smith, Jonathan M. "Warfighter Analytics Using Smartphones for Health (WASH)." https://www.darpa.mil/program/warfighter-analytics-using-smartphones-for-health.

Spitzer, Julie. "IBM's Watson recommended 'unsafe and incorrect' cancer treatments, STAT report finds." *Becker's Healthcare*, July 25, 2018. https://www.beckershospitalreview.com/artificial-intelligence/ibm-s-watson-recommended-unsafe-and-incorrect-cancer-treatments-stat-report-finds.html..

Strickland, Eliza. "How IBM Watson Overpromised and Underdelivered on AI Health Care." IEEE Spectrum: Technology, Engineering, and Science News. April 2, 2019. https://spectrum.ieee.org/biomedical/diagnostics/how-ibm-watson-overpromised-and-underdelivered-on-ai-health-care.

Tajitsu, Naomi. "Japanese Automakers Look to Robots to Aid the Elderly." *Scientific American*. April 12, 2017. https://www.scientificamerican.com/article/japanese-automakers-look-to-robots-to-aid-the-elderly/.

Tielman, Myrthe L., Mark A. Neerincx, Rafael Bidarra, Ben Kybartas, and Willem-Paul Brinkman. "A Therapy System for Post-Traumatic Stress Disorder Using a Virtual Agent and Virtual Storytelling to Reconstruct Traumatic Memories." Journal of Medical Systems 41, no. 8 (2017): 125.

Truschel, Jessica. "Top 25 Mental Health Apps for 2020: An Alternative to Therapy?" Psycom.net–Mental Health Treatment Resource Since 1986, March 19, 2020. https://www.psycom.net/25-best-mental-health-apps.

United States Bureau of Labor Statistics. "Home Health Aides and Personal Care Aides: Occupational Outlook Handbook," September 4, 2019. https://www.bls.gov/ooh/healthcare/home-health-aides-and-personal-care-aides.htm.

Vaidyam, Aditya, and John Torous. "Chatbots: What Are They and Why Care?" *Psychiatric Times*. June 27, 2019. https://www.psychiatrictimes.com/telepsychiatry/chatbots-what-are-they-and-why-care.

Vincent, James. "Twitter Taught Microsoft's Friendly AI Chatbot to Be a Racist Asshole in Less Than a Day." *The Verge*. March 24, 2016. https://www.theverge.com/2016/3/24/11297050/tay-microsoft-chatbot-racist.

Vincent, James. "Google's AI Thinks This Turtle Looks like a Gun, Which Is a Problem." *The Verge*. November 2, 2017. https://www.theverge.com/2017/11/2/16597276/google-ai-image-attacks-adversarial-turtle-rifle-3d-printed.

Yan, Alice. "How a Robot Passed China's Medical Licensing Exam." *South China Morning Post*, November 20, 2017. Accessed April 20, 2019.

Yu, V. L. "Antimicrobial Selection by a Computer. A Blinded Evaluation by Infectious Diseases Experts." *JAMA: The Journal of the American Medical Association* 242, no. 12 (1979): 1279–282.

La inteligencia artificial como médico clínico:
un argumento para el uso ético de futuras tecnologías en un entorno médico

Sara Gaines

En el mundo de hoy, la ciencia ficción se ha vuelto una realidad. La presencia de la inteligencia artificial (IA) en las sociedades de todo el mundo continúa creciendo, desde los dispositivos de bolsillo hasta el software globalizado. Un área en particular, la medicina, ha tomado debida nota de las formas en que dichas tecnologías han sido implementadas y de lo que se vislumbra en el horizonte. No es de extrañar que las tecnologías de la IA sean implementadas cada vez más en un entorno de atención médica y que una mayor implementación conlleva una mayor preocupación sobre el uso ético de la IA. Conforme ha avanzado la tecnología, siempre se han presentado dilemas éticos, pero existe un área en particular que pronto deberá estar en el centro de estos diálogos: la de la relación médico-paciente. El desarrollo y la aplicación de futuras tecnologías pueden situar a la IA en el rol de tomador de decisiones en cuestiones médicas, lo que probablemente pudiera influir en la relación médico-paciente. Una versión de esta tecnología, a la que me refiero como personal médico de IA de primera línea, puede implementarse de manera ética apegada a dos criterios. Primero, el personal médico de IA de primera línea debe utilizarse en entornos donde el uso de IA aligere la carga del sistema hospitalario y permita un mayor acceso a la atención médica. Segundo, dichas tecnologías deben implementarse en entornos donde los pacientes hayan demostrado la capacidad de conectarse a nivel personal con las tecnologías de la IA. En Estados Unidos, existe un sistema hospitalario donde podría implementarse la IA como médico de primera línea y a la vez apegarse a estos criterios: la Veterans Health Administration (Administración de Salud de los Veteranos).

Es imposible no considerar las futuras aplicaciones de la IA en la medicina cuando ya la sociedad ha adoptado la IA. El diccionario Oxford define inteligencia artificial como "la teoría y el desarrollo de sistemas informáticos capaces de realizar tareas que generalmente precisan de la inteligencia humana".[1] De acuerdo con esta definición, muchas de las tecnologías que la gente utiliza a diario indican qué tan relacionada está la IA con la vida de las personas en todo el mundo. Los teléfonos que llevamos en el bolsillo son capaces de buscar rápidamente, no sólo el lugar más cercano para comer con las mejores reseñas, sino también decirnos cómo llegar allí. Cada uno de nosotros ha buscado algún artículo en línea, solo para darse cuenta de que ese producto que ha sido anunciado en plataformas de redes sociales y en sitios web dista mucho de las primeras búsquedas en internet. Encontrar música nueva resulta más fácil que nunca con los servicios de streaming que sugieren algo nuevo todos los días. Estos son solo algunos ejemplos de IA que se han incorporado fácilmente a la vida cotidiana, pero conforme avance la tecnología, la presencia de la IA continuará incrementándose. Sin embargo, para estudiar el impacto de la integración de futuras tecnologías no solo en las actividades cotidianas, sino específicamente en un entorno de atención médica, es necesario tener una mayor claridad sobre la IA, que la definición que ofrece el diccionario.

Para distinguir mejor entre las tareas realizadas por el hombre y la tecnología "capaz de realizar tareas que generalmente precisan de la inteligencia humana", la IA ha avanzado a una fase en la que puede discutirse en términos de la IA débil y la IA fuerte. Las tecnologías de la IA que entran dentro de la categoría IA débil son aquellas que están estructuradas en torno a una sola capacidad humana.[2] Por ejemplo, el razonamiento probabilístico y la percepción visual. Por otra parte, la IA fuerte abarca tecnologías hipotéticas consideradas como equivalentes a la inteligencia humana e incluso sobrehumanas en términos de capacidad para ejecutar tareas inteligentes.[3] Las tecnologías IA fuertes serían aquellas que pueden entender el simbolismo, adaptarse a entornos sociales o concebir procesos de pensamiento ideológico propios. En muchos sentidos, esta división es sinónimo de las tecnologías actuales (débiles) y de las futuras tecnologías (fuertes). Sin embargo, dicha división no es binaria, sino que existe en una escala. Existen muchas tecnologías que sobrepasan los límites de los algoritmos de búsqueda o programas diseñados para encontrar la siguiente

---

1. Oxford English Dictionary Online, s.v. "artificial intelligence," [inteligencia artificial] Noviembre de 2019. Oxford: Oxford University Press. https://www.oed.com/view/Entry/271625?redirectedFrom=artificial+intelligence#eid.
2. Stuart J. Russell and Peter Norvig, *Artificial Intelligence a Modern Approach* [Inteligencia artificial, un enfoque modern] (Boston: Pearson, 2016)
3. Erik Brynjolfsson y Andrew McAfee, *The Second Machine Age: Work, Progress, and Prosperity in a Time of Brilliant Technologies* [La segunda era de las máquinas: trabajo, progreso y prosperidad en una época de tecnologías brillantes](Vancouver, BC: Langara College, 2018).

canción en su lista de reproducción y hacia lo que alguna vez y que todavía se considera de muchas maneras, posible solo en la ciencia ficción. Muchas de las ideas de IA de la ciencia ficción que se centran en tecnologías IA fuerte y en la manera cómo son representadas, pueden y han influido en gran medida en la percepción que se tiene de la IA en una sociedad. Dependiendo de la forma en que se represente a la IA en estos ejemplos ficticios, puede ya sea afectar o ayudar a que los seres humanos interactúen con las tecnologías en desarrollo.

Aunque ciertamente no sea el caso en todas las partes del mundo, Estados Unidos tiene un concepto dudoso de las tecnologías de la IA. La IA teórica capaz de pensar por sí misma ha sido ampliamente representada como villana en la cultura estadounidense. El temor a la IA en el mundo occidental fue documentado mucho antes de que la persona promedio comenzara a interactuar con la IA de forma cotidiana. Isaac Asimov publicó *Yo, Robot*, su colección de cuentos sobre robots equipados con IA y sobre cómo interactuaban con el mundo que les rodeaba, en el año de 1950. Entre estos cuentos se encuentran las famosas tres leyes de la robótica:

1. Un robot no puede hacerle daño a un ser humano o, por inacción, permitir que un ser humano sufra daño.
2. Un robot debe obedecer las órdenes dictadas por los seres humanos, excepto cuando tales órdenes entren en conflicto con la Primera Ley.
• Un robot debe proteger su propia existencia siempre y cuando esto no entre en conflicto con la Primera o la Segunda Ley.[4]

Estas leyes, aunque adaptadas y ampliadas por diversos autores, incluso por el propio Asimov, en el transcurso de las siguientes décadas han influido considerablemente no solo en la ciencia ficción, sino también en el campo de la ética de la Inteligencia Artificial. Gran parte de la ficción que estudia el avance de las tecnologías de la IA se funda en lo que sucede cuando estas leyes se llevan al extremo, o incluso se quebrantan, y la IA que estaba originalmente destinada a ayudar a la humanidad se convierte en el enemigo. En el sentido más básico, gran parte de la cultura desarrollada alrededor de las tecnologías de IA en los Estados Unidos es la del miedo.

Uno de los ejemplos más famosos de este miedo tiene lugar en la franquicia *Terminator*, en donde cada punto de la trama gira en torno a la derrota de Skynet, una superinteligencia artificial autoconsciente (el punto más alto en

---

4. Isaac Asimov, "Círculo vicioso" *Yo, Robot*. Greenwich, CT: Fawcett Publications, 1950.

la escala de la IA fuerte). En 1984 se vio el lanzamiento de la primera de seis películas y para el 2010, toda la franquicia comprendía películas, programas de televisión, videojuegos, historietas, parques temáticos y probablemente todas las formas de mercancía imaginables habían recaudado ganancias por más de tres mil millones de dólares.[5] Desde entonces se han estrenado dos películas más de la franquicia. A la población estadounidense le atrae la idea de que una IA, en este caso Skynet, sea malvada. Y no es solo la franquicia *Terminator* la que generó un gran fanatismo a partir de esta idea, la franquicia *The Matrix* constituye otro elemento básico de la cultura pop estadounidense de miles de millones de dólares que gira en torno a la historia de la caída de la sociedad humana ante la insubordinación de la IA. Junto con estas dos franquicias surgen innumerables películas, series de televisión y libros que protagonizan sistemas de IA malvada. El tropo es tan popular en los medios de comunicación estadounidenses que las listas de las "IA asesinas" favoritas incluyen ítems de todo tipo, desde la cruda ciencia ficción hasta dibujos animados infantiles.[6]

Esta visión de la IA no es igual en todo el mundo. La visión de las tecnologías de la IA en Japón se opone casi por completo a la del miedo a la IA presente en la cultura popular de Estados Unidos. Los medios de comunicación japoneses representan ampliamente a los robots y a las tecnologías de la IA fuerte como si fueran amigos e incluso en muchos casos, amantes.[7] Este enfoque tan distinto de la IA ha sido atribuido a una diferencia de la cultura en general derivada del distinto marco religioso propio del Japón.[8] La historia del budismo y del sintoísmo en el Japón ha llevado a la sociedad a pensar en todas las cosas, tanto sintientes como no sintientes, como si fueran dignas de respeto, en vez de las nociones judeo-cristianas donde

5. Business Wire, "Pacificor Names Latham & Watkins to Field Terminator Inquiries," [Pacificor nombra a Latham & Watkins para atender las inquietudes sobre Terminator] *Berkshire Hathaway*, 17 de febrero de 2010, https://web.archive.org/web/20170306034914/ http://www.businesswire.com/news/home/20100217005514/en/Pacificor-Names-Latham-Watkins-Field-Terminator-Inquiries.
6. Andrew Dyce, "Our 10 Favorite Killer A.I.'s in Movies", *Screen Rant*, 18 de abril de 2014. https://screenrant.com/artificial-intelligence-movies-evil-computers/.
7. Cat Ana, "Why the Japanese Find Deep Love with Deep Learning"[Por qué los japoneses encuentran el amor profundo con el aprendizaje profundo], *Medium* (*Becoming Human: Artificial Intelligence Magazine*, 12 de febrero de 2019), https://becominghuman.ai/why-the-japanese-find-deep-love-with-deep-learning-829e1bb629c2.
8. Joi Ito, "Why Westerners Fear Robots and the Japanese Do Not" [Por qué los occidentales temen a los robots y los japoneses no], *Wired* (Conde Nast, 30 de julio de 2018), https://www.wired.com/story/ideas-joi-ito-robot-overlords/.

la jerarquía humana está por encima de todo, excepto de Dios.[9] Gracias a esta capacidad para apreciar la vida en todas las cosas, la sociedad japonesa pudo apreciar la vida en la IA y en la robótica, lo que la llevó rápidamente a considerar estas tecnologías como los amigos y amantes representados en sus medios de comunicación. Incluso en diálogos sobre las tecnologías de la IA médica observadas en Japón, la tendencia para aceptar dicha tecnología se atribuye directamente a la caricatura de la década de 1950 Astro Boy.[10]

A diferencia de la amabilidad de la IA que se aprecia en Japón, las advertencias sobre la IA inherentes a la cultura popular estadounidense no son sutiles. Existe una sensación de inevitabilidad, en estas franquicias masivas, de que un día la ciencia vaya demasiado lejos y que la IA destinada a ser útil, se vuelva un día en contra de la humanidad sin importar si las Tres Leyes forman parte de su código o si se toman otras medidas de seguridad. No es de extrañar que una búsqueda académica en línea de las palabras clave "inteligencia artificial" y "demasiado lejos" dentro de las publicaciones occidentales arroje más de 39 mil resultados.[11] Sin embargo, estos temores no han desalentado el avance de las tecnologías de la IA en el mundo real. Dicho desarrollo no siempre ha sido exitoso, pero cada intento fallido constituye un paso más hacia al éxito.

En un "simple" intento por crear una IA que funcionara tan bien como una presencia humana en las redes sociales, Microsoft descubrió rápidamente que su bot no estaba a la altura de las circunstancias. La inteligencia artificial, Tay, fue dada a conocer vía Twitter en el año 2016 con su propia cuenta, pero el experimento fue suspendido después de tan solo dieciséis horas, el tiempo suficiente para que Tay pasara de ser una simpática chatbot a usar insultos racistas.[12] El software de reconocimiento facial, a pesar de ser una versión de la IA que muchos de nosotros usamos en los actuales teléfonos celulares, también ha demostrado ser menos confiable cuando se implementa a gran escala. Por ejemplo, el intento a gran escala en China, de multar a peatones

---

9. Joi Ito, "Why Westerners."
10. Don Lee, "Desperate for Workers, Aging Japan Turns to Robots for Healthcare", [Desesperado por conseguir trabajadores, el Japón senescente recurre a los robots para el cuidado de la salud] *Los Angeles Times*, 25 de julio de 2019, https://www.latimes.com/world-nation/story/2019-07-25/desperate-for-workers-aging-japan-turns-to-robots-for-healthcare.
11. Resultados de una búsqueda en Google Scholar el 11 de abril de 2020, excluyendo patentes y citas.
12. James Vincent, "Twitter Taught Microsoft's Friendly AI Chatbot to Be a Racist Asshole in Less Than a Day." [Twitter le enseñó al amistoso chatbot de inteligencia artificial de Microsoft a ser un gilipollas racista en menos de un día] *The Verge*. 24 de marzo de 2016. https://www.theverge.com/2016/3/24/11297050/tay-microsoft-chatbot-racist.

imprudentes en pro de la seguridad pública terminó con la rápida acumulación de multas a modelos y actores cuyos rostros se anunciaban en la parte lateral de las unidades de transporte público.[13] Algunas tecnologías de identificación no especializada tampoco han logrado los mejores resultados cuando se trata de identificar un solo objeto en vez de un rostro. En un ejemplo, una tortuga fue confundida con un arma.[14] Sin embargo, por cada uno de estos fallos documentados, se da un paso hacia el progreso.

En los últimos años, las tecnologías de IA que parecían surgidas de una novela de ciencia ficción y que se acercaban más a lo que se consideraría una IA fuerte han tenido gran éxito. Pudiera ser que la IA de Google haya confundido una tortuga con un arma, pero se dispone de muchas aplicaciones especializadas en la identificación de objetos que son capaces de permitir que el usuario promedio identifique incluso especies de animales o vegetales raros que haya a su alrededor.[15] El avance de la IA ha tenido un impacto no solo en los animales que hay en el patio; para detener el avance de las actividades de caza furtiva en África, se utilizan drones equipados con IA.[16] Las ciudades también han comenzado a buscar formas de resolver su problemática actual, a través de IA. La ciudad de Los Ángeles ha recurrido a la IA como un recurso para resolver su añejo y vulnerable sistema de tuberías.[17] La IA pudiera no ser perfecta en todos los sentidos y que sea necesario un mayor desarrollo para evitar errores tan graves como el del bot Tay, sin embargo, las tecnologías de IA del usuario han logrado

13. Melanie Ehrenkranz, "Facial Recognition Flags Woman on Bus Ad for 'Jaywalking' in China"[El reconocimiento facial identifica a mujer en anuncio de autobús por 'cruzar de manera imprudente' en China"]. *Gizmodo* 26 de noviembre de 2018. https://gizmodo.com/facial-recognition-flags-woman-on-bus-ad-for-jaywalking-1830654750.

14. James Vincent, "Google's AI Thinks This Turtle Looks like a Gun, Which Is a Problem." [La IA de Google cree que esta tortuga parece un arma, lo cual es un problema], *The Verge*. 2 de noviembre de 2017. https://www.theverge.com/2017/11/2/16597276/google-ai-image-attacks-adversarial-turtle-rifle-3d-printed.

15. Emily Matchar, "AI Plant and Animal Identification Helps Us All Be Citizen Scientists"[La identificación de plantas y animals gracias a la inteligencia artificial nos ayuda a convertirnos en ciudadanos científicos], Smithsonian.com (Smithsonian Institution, 7 de junio de 2017), https://www.smithsonianmag.com/innovation/ai-plant-and-animal-identification-helps-us-all-be-citizen-scientists-180963525/.

16. Builddie, "The Role of Artificial Intelligence in Wildlife Conservation"[El rol de la inteligencia artificial en la conservación de la vida silvestre], *Medium*, 15 de mayo de 2019, https://medium.com/builddie/the-role-of-artificial-intelligence-in-wildlife-conservation-5dc3af2b4222.

17. Gary Polakovic, "The next Big Effort in AI: Keeping L.A.'s Water Flowing Post-Earthquake"[El siguiente gran esfuerzo de la IA: mantener el flujo del agua en L.A. después del temblor], *USC News*, 4 de octubre de 2019, https://news.usc.edu/160680/ai-la-water-supply-earthquake-usc-research/.

tener éxito. En el campo de la medicina, la historia de la IA desarrollada últimamente no es la excepción. Aunque algunos intentos han tenido más éxito que otros, la tecnología, en un sentido amplio, ha continuado avanzando. A través de este desarrollo, el uso de IA en un entorno médico ha planteado dilemas éticos, incluso cuando ha tenido éxito la utilización de algunas de las tecnologías de IA. Dichos dilemas solo se han incrementado conforme la IA se acerca más hacia al lado de la IA fuerte y los sistemas de la IA comienzan a intercalarse en espacios que antes eran exclusivos para los médicos humanos. En esta intercalación existe la inquietud de que la IA reemplace a un médico, quebrantando así la ética establecida dentro del firme y arraigado marco del principialismo, el marco ético de mayor prevalencia en el campo de la medicina moderna, particularmente en Estados Unidos.

El ensayo de Beauchamp y Childress sobre el principialismo detalla un marco ético basado en la forma de interacción del médico con el paciente. Los cuatro principios (no maleficencia, beneficencia, justicia y autonomía) guían la forma en que el médico debe interactuar con el paciente, apoyarlo o proveerle.[18] Esta relación entre médico y paciente es, por lo tanto, clave para la práctica ética de la medicina. Cuando se establece la relación médico-paciente, se crea un sentido de confiabilidad.[19] Según Los principios de la ética biomédica, "nada es más importante para las organizaciones de atención médica que el mantener una cultura de confianza".[20] La literatura que se aborda posteriormente en el presente ensayo indica que el temor a introducir la IA en el campo de la medicina gira en torno a cuestiones de confianza, las cuales podrían reducirse al temor de que el paciente no pudiera confiar en ningún diagnóstico, tratamiento o interacción con alguna entidad de IA. Estas inquietudes han surgido a lo largo de la historia de la IA en la medicina, comenzando con los primeros programas de investigación.

En la década de 1970, el campo de la medicina dejó entrever por vez primera la implementación de tecnologías de la IA. El MYCIN, un incipiente sistema de IA diseñado por investigadores de la Escuela de Medicina de Stanford, fue utilizado para identificar ciertas bacterias como la de la meningitis y la bacteriemia y sugerir opciones de tratamiento para prevenir

---

18. Thomas L. Beauchamp and James F. Childress, *Principles of Biomedical Ethics* [Principios de *ética* biomédica]. New York: Oxford University Press, 2013.
19. Mark A. Hall et al., "Trust in Physicians and Medical Institutions: What Is It, Can It Be Measured, and Does It Matter?," [La confianza en los medicos e instituciones médicas: ¿qué es? ¿puede medirse? y ¿por qué importa?] *The Milbank Quarterly* 79, no. 4 (2001): 613.
20. Beauchamp y Childress, *Principles* [Principios], 40.

infecciones graves.[21] Toda una década antes de la invención del Internet, el MYCIN fue capaz de crear un plan de tratamiento con un índice de aceptabilidad del 65% según los parámetros del estudio. En comparación, se les pidió a cinco profesores que crearan un plan de tratamiento basado en los mismos datos y los índices de aceptabilidad asignadas a esos planes quedaron entre 42.5 y 62.5%. Incluso con resultados tan prometedores, la ética con respecto al uso del MYCIN fue puesta de inmediato en tela de juicio ya que se había elaborado un plan de tratamiento individualizado mediante un modelo de probabilidad, en vez de hacerlo con un médico real.[22] En resumen, ¿cómo podría una máquina elaborar un plan preciso si no existía una relación con el paciente con el fin de determinar qué plan de tratamiento sería efectivo? Aunque el MYCIN nunca se implementó en un entorno médico, estas preocupaciones iniciales persistieron conforme avanzaba la IA y empezaba a ganar terreno en los entornos médicos.

Los intentos más actuales para integrar la IA a la medicina occidental pueden encontrarse en los sistemas de apoyo a las decisiones clínicas (CDSS, por sus siglas en inglés) y de manera específica en los sistemas para la toma de decisiones de diagnóstico (DDSS, por sus siglas en inglés). El propósito detrás de un DDSS es interpretar datos con el fin de ayudar a los médicos. La asistencia que se brinda a través de un DDSS puede, en teoría, ayudar a que el médico brinde un mejor diagnóstico sobre un problema de salud identificando las situaciones y señales de alerta de condiciones que se estén desarrollando con el fin de que las revise.[23] Hasta hoy, el campo en donde el DDSS ha tenido mayor impacto, ha sido la imagenología, debido a la aplicación de la tecnología a los sistemas de radiología médica como las resonancias magnéticas y las tomografías computarizadas. Los métodos tradicionales de evaluación de imágenes médicas pueden dar lugar a diagnósticos equivocados, haciendo necesaria una segunda opinión, lo que puede en ocasiones, complicar aún

---

21. V. L. Yu, "Antimicrobial Selection by a Computer. A Blinded Evaluation by Infectious Diseases Experts," [Selección de antimicrobianos por computadora. Una evaluación ciega realizada por expertos en enfermedades infecciosas] *JAMA: The Journal of the American Medical Association* 242, no. 12 (1979): 1279–282.
22. David E. Heckerman y Edward H. Shortliffe, "From Certainty Factors to Belief Networks" [De los factores de certeza a las redes de las creencias], *Artificial Intelligence in Medicine* 4, no. 1 (1992): 37.
23. Eta S. Berner y Tonya J. La Lande, "Overview of Clinical Decision Support Systems" [Panorama general de los sistemas de soporte a las decisiones clínicas], en *Clinical Decision Support Systems: Theory and Practice*, ed. Eta S. Berner (Suiza: Springer International Press, 2016), 3.

más el asunto.[24] Además, estos métodos también dejan a los médicos cada vez más agotados al final de la jornada laboral, lo que se traduce en diagnósticos menos precisos durante la misma.[25] Los DDSS que ya se han desarrollado y los que se vislumbran en el horizonte de la implementación en el campo de la medicina, están destinados a contrarrestar algunos de estos problemas al brindar una segunda opinión en tiempo real. El DDSS puede hacer sugerencias de manera inmediata en estos casos, pero es el médico quien toma la decisión final sobre el diagnóstico y el tratamiento.

Basándose en el entusiasmo que existe en torno a la idea de que el DDSS se integre por completo al campo de la medicina, la compañía IBM presentó lo que posiblemente sea uno de los ejemplos más famosos de la IA que se hayan utilizado en diagnósticos médicos: Watson for Oncology (Watson para oncología). El Watson de IBM, es un ordenador con la capacidad de entender el lenguaje y contenidos naturales que fue desarrollado mucho más allá de su propósito original de introducir la tecnología al campo de la medicina.[26] Watson fue originalmente diseñado para competir contra concursantes humanos en el programa de televisión *Jeopardy* y que al final obtuvo el éxito, venciendo en el año 2011 a Ken Jennings, el "más grande participante de todos los tiempos", del programa *Jeopardy*".[27] Después de dicha victoria pública para las tecnologías de la IA, IBM redirigió el enfoque de Watson hacia la medicina, lanzando finalmente a Watson for Oncology en el año 2016.[28] Publicitado como la siguiente frontera de la medicina, Watson fue representado como un sistema de IA capaz, no solo de ayudar

24. Christopher Eakins et al., "Second Opinion Interpretations by Specialty Radiologists at a Pediatric Hospital: Rate of Disagreement and Clinical Implications,"[Interpretaciones de segundas opiniones por radiólogos especializados en un hospital pediátrico: tasa de desacuerdo e implicaciones clínicas] *American Journal of Roentgenology* 199, no. 4 (2012): pp. 916-920.

25. Elizabeth A. Krupinski et al., "Long Radiology Workdays Reduce Detection and Accommodation Accuracy," [Las largas jornadas de trabajo en radiología reducen la precisión de la detección y el acomodo] *Journal of the American College of Radiology* 7, no. 9 (2010): pp. 698–704

26. IBM, "Watson Overview"[Panorama general de Watson], The DeepQA Research Team, 25 de julio de 2016, https://researcher.watson.ibm.com/researcher/view_group.php?id=2099.

27. Eric Brown, "Watson: The *Jeopardy*! Challenge and beyond "[Watson: *Jeopardy*, el reto y más allá], 2013 *IEEE 12th International Conference on Cognitive Informatics and Cognitive Computing*, 2013.

28. Sala de prensa de IBM, "Manipal Hospitals Announces National Launch of IBM Watson for Oncology"[*Manipal Hospitals* anuncia el lanzamiento a nivel nacional de *Watson for Oncology* de IBM], 26 de julio de 2016, https://www-03.ibm.com/press/in/en/pressrelease/50290.wss.

en la interpretación de imágenes diagnósticas, sino también de suministrar planes de tratamiento reales y efectivos sin la aprobación de un médico. Los defensores de la IA consideraban que Watson for Oncology era una forma de demostrar los beneficios de introducir una IA más avanzada al área de la medicina, pero a pesar de esto, predominaron las cuestiones éticas con respecto a que una máquina tomara decisiones médicas.[29] Como posteriormente se diera a conocer mediante mensajes internos de IBM hechos públicos en julio de 2018, muchas de estas inquietudes con respecto al uso de Watson for Oncology tenían fundamento.

Un informe de la empresa STAT reveló que los ejecutivos de IBM estaban muy conscientes de los problemas que se encontraron dentro de los sistemas de Watson for Oncology, destacando que Watson proporcionó "numerosos ejemplos de recomendaciones de tratamientos inseguros e incorrectos".[30] Muchos de estos problemas ya eran del conocimiento de los empleados de IBM. Los registros muestran que IBM trató de ponerse en contacto con los médicos para informarles sobre las "muy limitadas" habilidades de Watson.[31] La mayoría de estos intentos fracasó y los sistemas hospitalarios continuaron operando bajo el supuesto de que Watson suministraba las opciones de tratamiento adecuado para los pacientes. Después de que se publicara el informe STAT y salieran a la luz los inseguros planes de tratamiento de Watson, muchos sistemas hospitalarios se apresuraron a emitir declaraciones para mitigar el temor de que la AI había ido demasiado lejos y reemplazado a los médicos en cuanto a la toma de decisiones médicas. En una declaración que aseguraba al público que Watson se había utilizado únicamente como herramienta y no para la toma de decisiones, el portavoz de un hospital comentó: "Ninguna tecnología puede reemplazar a un médico ni el conocimiento que éste tiene sobre el paciente como persona".[32] El mensaje era claro: la relación médico-paciente no se había debilitado por

---

29. Jennifer Bresnick, "Artificial Intelligence in Healthcare Market to See 40% CAGR Surge" [La inteligencia artificial en el mercado de la atención médica verá un aumento del 40 % de la tasa compuesta de crecimiento anual], HealthITAnalytics, 24 de julio de 2017, https://healthitanalytics.com/news/artificial-intelligence-in-healthcare-market-to-see-40-cagr-surge.
30. Casey Ross and Ike Swetlitz, "IBM's Watson supercomputer recommended 'unsafe and incorrect' cancer treatments, internal documents show," *STAT*, 25 de julio de 2018.
31. Julie Spitzer, "IBM 's Watson recommended' unsafe and incorrect 'cancer treatments, STAT report findings," [La supercomputadora Watson de IBM recomendó tratamientos contra el cáncer "inseguros e incorrectos", según muestran documentos internos] *Becker's Healthcare*, 25 de julio de 2018.
32. Spitzer, "IBM 's Watson" [Watson de IBM].

el uso de Watson for Oncology ya que los médicos no estaban en realidad, utilizando el sistema de la IA para tomar decisiones importantes; esas decisiones las tomaron exclusivamente los médicos. Sin embargo, incluso después de que se cuestionara la exactitud de las decisiones oncológicas de Watson, el programa de software continúa siendo implementado en los sistemas de atención médica actuales, incluyendo al menos setenta de los Centros Médicos de Asuntos de los Veteranos (VAMC, por sus siglas en inglés) en Estados Unidos.[33]

El uso continuo de Watson for Oncology no es la única señal de que los sistemas de atención médica continúan estando interesados en explorar el funcionamiento de la IA en el campo de la medicina. En efecto, el diagnóstico asistido por IA ha sido implementado a la par con la garantía de que es el médico quien tiene en realidad la última palabra, pero existen empresas en todo el mundo que están desarrollando tecnologías de IA que se adentran más en el ámbito médico. Hasta hoy, de hecho, han surgido preocupaciones muy serias sobre si la IA reemplazará a los médicos.[34] Actualmente existen numerosos programas que han podido aprobar con éxito los exámenes del consejo médico.

El primer país que vio a una IA aprobar un examen de licencia médica fue China, en el año 2017. El robot equipado con IA, Xiaoyi, que en mandarín significa "pequeño médico", acaparó la primera plana al obtener 456 de los 600 puntos en el examen de licencia médica en China, o sea, 96 puntos arriba de la calificación mínima aprobatoria.[35] Es importante considerar que este examen chino no puede aprobarse solo con memorización repetitiva. El examen está estructurado de manera que los aspirantes a médicos deben estudiar los casos y determinar la respuesta apropiada en función de la información proporcionada, demostrando así que son capaces de interpretar la información que se les presenta y tomar una decisión

---

33. Eliza Strickland, "How IBM Watson Overpromised and Underd delivered on AI Health Care"[Cómo Watson de IBM prometió de más e incumplió como IA de cuidado medico], *IEEE Spectrum: Technology, Engineering, and Science News*, 2 de abril de 2019, https://spectrum.ieee.org/biomedical/diagnostics/how-ibm-watson-overpromised-and-underdided-on-ai-health-care.

34. Kyle E. Karches, "Against the iDoctor: Why Artificial Intelligence Should Not Replace Physician Judgment"[Contra el iDoctor: por qué la inteligencia artificial no debería reemplazar al criterio del médico], *Theoretical Medicine and Bioethics* 39 (2): 92

35. Ma Si y Cheng Yu, "Chinese Robot Becomes World 's First Machine to Pass Medical Exam"[Robot chino se convierte en la primera máquina del mundo en aprobar un examen médico], *China Daily*, 10 de noviembre de 2017, http://www.chinadaily.com.cn/business/tech/2017-11/10/content_34362656.htm.

informada y fundamentada.[36] El primer intento de Xiaoyi por aprobar el examen, brinda una pauta sobre la dificultad del mismo, puesto que la IA solo obtuvo una calificación un poco mayor de 100 puntos. Antes de su siguiente intento, el equipo de investigación hizo que Xiaoyi "estudiara" facilitándole al robot una gran cantidad de libros de texto y archivos de casos médicos.[37] Al igual que todos los demás médicos que aprobaron el examen en ese entonces, Xiaoyi necesitaba aprender para poder aprobar el examen escrito. Sin embargo, cuando Xiaoyi demostró que la IA era toda una conocedora de las enfermedades médicas, el equipo de investigación se apresuró a anunciar que Xiaoyi solo podía "hacer sugerencias a los médicos para ayudarlos a identificar problemas más rápidamente y evitar algunos riesgos".[38] A pesar de que la IA aprobó un examen de licencia, aún era necesario aclarar que los pacientes recibirían atención por parte de médicos humanos y no de una IA.

Se percibió una reacción muy diferente la siguiente vez que una IA aprobó un examen del consejo médico. En junio de 2018, la IA de Babylon Health aprobó el examen de membresía del Reino Unido del Colegio Real de Médicos Generales (MRCGP, por sus siglas en inglés). El MRCGP es el último de una serie de exámenes destinados a poner a prueba el conocimiento de los estudiantes de medicina en el campo al que están ansiosos por ingresar. En resumen, la aprobación del MRCGP significa que un estudiante de medicina, después de muchos años de estudio, está finalmente preparado para ejercer la medicina de forma independiente. La puntuación promedio entre el 2012 y el 2017 fue del 72% La IA de la compañía Babylon obtuvo un 81%.[39] En una declaración publicada tras el éxito de la IA de Babylon, el fundador y director general de Babylon, el doctor Ali Parsa, no aseguró a la gente que dicha tecnología no reemplazaría a los médicos o que no era capaz de tomar decisiones médicas directamente con un paciente. De hecho, señaló lo contrario. Al resaltar que existen muchas áreas donde la posibilidad de ver a un médico es extremadamente

---

36. Alice Yan, "How a Robot Passed China 's Medical Licensing Exam"[Cómo un robot aprobó el examen de licencia médica en China], *South China Morning Post*, 20 de noviembre de 2017, consultado el 20 de abril de 2019.
37. Si and Yu, "Chinese Robot."
38. Yan, "How a Robot."
39. Babylon Health, "Babylon AI Achieves Equivalent Accuracy with Human Doctors in Global Healthcare First," [La IA de Babylon logra una precision equiparable con la de los médicos humanos en Global Healthcare First] *PR Newswire: News Distribution, Targeting and Monitoring*, 27 de junio de 2018.

limitada y los sistemas de atención médica están saturados, el doctor Parsa afirmó que la aprobación exitosa del examen MRCGP por parte de la IA "mostraba claramente cómo los servicios de salud expandidos gracias a la IA podían disminuir la carga de los sistemas de atención médica en todo el mundo".[40] El cambio de narrativa queda claro con el éxito de la IA de Babylon; puede ser que el futuro rol de la IA en la medicina no sea el de una herramienta de consulta para los médicos, sino que muy bien podría actuar como un médico en sí.

Los cambios recientes en el campo de la medicina han demostrado que muy bien podría aprobarse la visión del doctor Parsa para el futuro uso de la IA. Actualmente, un área de la medicina con un crecimiento exponencial es la telemedicina, y ese crecimiento da pie a diálogos en torno a la naturaleza cambiante sobre cómo se administran los medicamentos a los pacientes.[41] En Estados Unidos, las opciones de telesalud, definida en un estudio como "videoconferencia, monitoreo a distancia, consultas electrónicas y comunicaciones inalámbricas", fue puesta a disposición de los pacientes a través de sistemas hospitalarios que aumentaron del 35 al 76% entre los años 2010 y 2017.[42] Un aspecto común de la telemedicina es la opción de citas virtuales como las que se ofrecen a través de la Cleveland Clinic, con el propósito de tratar enfermedades básicas de primera línea tales como el resfriado común, las alergias e incluso la gripe, que no precisan necesariamente de que un paciente se reúna con un médico en persona, exactamente el tipo de cita al que se refiere el doctor Parsa de Babylon en su declaración sobre las posibles aplicaciones de la IA de Babylon.[43]

La gente en Estados Unidos ha empezado a sentirse más cómoda buscando orientación y tratamiento médicos a través de la tecnología. En todo el país y en el mundo existen ejemplos que demuestran que las personas no solamente están dispuestas a atenderse con un ser humano a través de la tecnología, sino que también podrían estar dispuestos a considerar las tecnologías de IA como si fuera un sustituto del médico. Uno de los ejemplos más destacados en la práctica médica actual es el uso de chatbots de terapia. Se ha demostrado que estos chatbots ayudan a los pacientes a

40. Babylon Health, "Babylon AI Achieves Equivalent Accuracy with Human Doctors."

41. Tommaso Iannitti et al., "Narrative Review of Telemedicine Consultation in Medical Practice" [Revisión narrativa de la consulta de telemedicina en la práctica médica", *Patient Preference and Adherence*, 2015, 65.

42. American Hospital Association, "Fact Sheet: Telehealth" [Hoja de datos: Telesalud], febrero de 2019.

43. "Cleveland Clinic Express Care® Online", Cleveland Clinic, 2019.

entender mejor su diagnóstico, así como para seguir su plan de tratamiento.[44] Otro estudio mostró que los pacientes que sufrían de estrés postraumático eran más abiertos y capaces de reconocer su trauma cuando le confiaban sus síntomas a un chatbot que cuando acudían a una cita en persona.[45] Sin embargo, esta versión particular de la IA en la medicina no significa que esté lista para reemplazar nuestros actuales modelos de terapia.

Si bien los participantes de estos estudios han estado dispuestos a conversar con un chatbot y han revelado más información de la que en un principio hubieran dado en una cita de terapia en persona o en una videollamada, la investigación ha mostrado que puede haber ciertas salvedades. Algunos de estos estudios indican de manera particular, que algunas personas están dispuestas a revelar más información a un chatbot solo después de saber que un médico humano va a volver a leer la transcripción posteriormente.[46] Dicho esto, aunque estos participantes se reconfortaron al saber que cualquier diagnóstico psicológico definitivo o retroalimentación terapéutica provendría de un médico humano, estuvieron dispuestos a seguir trabajando con una IA durante el inicio del proceso del tratamiento para esa determinada sesión. Y considerando el éxito comercial de las apps de terapia y el hecho de que la Asociación Americana de Psiquiatría haya comenzado a rastrear y a evaluar la posible eficacia de dichas apps, que a menudo cuentan con el componente de chatbot, existen muy pocas razones para pensar que la gente no utilizará más esta tecnología en el futuro.[47]

La idea de un terapeuta virtual plantea una dinámica diferente a la del modelo tradicional, incluso con la presencia de un médico humano al final del proceso. Con este nuevo modelo, la relación médico-paciente comienza a verse diferente de las interacciones presenciales, de un ser humano a otro, descritas por Beauchamp y Childress. Aunque los participantes quisieran

---

44. Aditya Vaidyam y John Torous. "Chatbots: What Are They and Why Care?" [Chatbots: ¿Qué son y por qué importan?] *Psychiatric Times*, 27 de junio de 2019. https://www.psychiatrictimes.com/telepsychiatry/chatbots-what-are-they-and-why-care.

45. Myrthe L. Tielman et al., "A Therapy System for Post-Traumatic Stress Disorder Using a Virtual Agent and Virtual Storytelling to Reconstruct Traumatic Memories" [Un sistema de terapia para el trastorno de estrés postraumático utilizando un agente y narración virtuales para reconstruir recuerdos traumáticos], *Journal of Medical Systems* 41, no. 8 (2017): 125.

46. Timothy W. Bickmore et al., "Response to a Relational Agent by Hospital Patients with Depressive Symptoms" [La respuesta a un agente relacional de pacientes hospitalizados con síntomas depresivos], *Interacting with Computers* 22, no. 4 (2010): 289.

47. Jessica Truschel, "Top 25 Mental Health Apps for 2020: An Alternative to Therapy?," [Las 25 mejores aplicaciones telefónicas de salud mental para 2020: ¿una alternativa a la terapia?] Psycom.net– Mental Health Treatment Resource Since 1986, 19 de marzo de 2020, https://www.psycom.net/25-best-mental-health-apps.

todavía estar seguros de que fuera un ser humano quien tomara la decisión final, el establecimiento inicial de la relación no fue con un ser humano, sino más bien con una IA. Lo anterior marca una divergencia de las actitudes que se han visto con respecto a las DDSS como Watson for Oncology que funcionan tras bambalinas. Esos sistemas de IA están diseñados para utilizarse como herramientas tras bambalinas en conjunto con la experiencia de un médico. Un chatbot virtual diseñado para brindar terapia interactúa primero con el ser humano y transmite posteriormente, la información recopilada de un ser humano a otro. Estas IA de chatbot no leen imágenes más bien funcionan con el diálogo y establecen una relación con el cliente. Pudiera ser que la relación no tenga un parecido directo como con la relación médico-paciente desarrollada por la medicina moderna, pero en estas circunstancias, la IA se está entrelazando indiscutiblemente en la relación entre un paciente y un médico. Y aunque los chatbots mencionados no pueden, obviamente, reemplazar la interacción presencial con un médico, se están desarrollando otras tecnologías a nivel mundial que, de igual manera, comienzan a trascender ese límite.

En Japón, donde ya se ve con buenos ojos la IA, las tecnologías de la IA que ayudan a los pacientes de manera directa han ido un paso más allá comparadas con los terapeutas en línea. Japón ha comenzado a implementar robots de atención primaria equipados con IA capaces de suministrar la dosis correcta de medicamentos y de atender las necesidades básicas de su población senescente en formas tan sencillas como la de ajustar la temperatura de sus habitaciones.[48] La demanda por la robótica se ha incrementado a tal grado en el campo de la atención geriátrica que muchos fabricantes de automóviles han rechazado el diseño de vehículos autónomos y, en cambio, proporcionan tecnologías como camas que se transforman en sillas de ruedas o piernas cibernéticas que permiten que los trabajadores en el área de la salud levanten por sí solos a pacientes pesados.[49] De manera más directa y personal, los robots humanoides equipados con IA, como Pepper de la empresa SoftBank Robotics, también han sido desarrollados para cantarle a los pacientes de edad avanzada, así como para responder preguntas básicas como "¿dónde queda el baño?"[50] Incluso los animales de

48. Naomi Tajitsu, "Japanese Automakers Look to Robots to Help the Elderly," [Fabricantes de automóviles japoneses recurren a robots para ayudar a los adultos mayores] *Scientific American*. 12 de abril de 2017, https://www.scientificamerican.com/article/japanese-automakers-look-to-robots-to-aid-the-elderly.
49. Don Lee, "Desperate for Workers."
50. Don Lee, "Desperate for Workers."

compañía de diseño japonés, como la foca robot Paro, han sido creados explícitamente para reaccionar ante la interacción humana y proporcionar los medios para que los pacientes de edad avanzada establezcan una relación con una entidad inanimada.[51]

Las tecnologías como Paro y Pepper están diseñadas deliberadamente para capitalizar la distintiva capacidad cultural para que los pacientes japoneses se conecten con la IA, gracias a la cual han tenido un gran éxito. Considerando esta capacidad de los individuos japoneses de ver a la IA de manera positiva, como se discutió previamente, no es de extrañar que estén a la vanguardia de adoptar IA en un entorno de atención médica. En estos ejemplos, la tecnología fue implementada para satisfacer las necesidades de la población senescente de Japón al atender la falta de trabajadores de cuidado médico disponibles. Al utilizar la tecnología de IA en ese entorno, los robots humanoides de IA japonesa cumplen con el primer requisito para la implementación de IA en un entorno de atención médica de manera ética. El segundo requisito de garantizar la capacidad para mantener la relación médico-paciente se cumple parcialmente, ya que los pacientes han demostrado una clara capacidad de identificarse con estas tecnologías, pero no de la misma manera en que un paciente y su médico tomarían decisiones. Si bien la IA humanoide en Japón no alcanza completamente los niveles de la tecnología del futuro que podrían llegar a implementarse dentro de un entorno de atención médica, estas tecnologías actuales constituyen, sin duda, un paso más en esa dirección.

Estados Unidos en general, podría no estar listo para la implementación a gran escala de una robótica humanoide equipada con IA como las que se aprecian en Japón. Más bien, una tecnología de IA que se adapte de manera más realista a los sistemas de salud de Estados Unidos, sería algo parecido a la IA de la empresa Babylon, donde la IA actúa como un médico de primera línea. Como tal, la IA diagnosticaría rápidamente enfermedades básicas como resfriados y gripe, y referiría a un médico o especialista humano cuando fuera necesario. Una IA de tal alcance podría implementarse en Estados Unidos siempre que se apegue a los dos requisitos éticos de satisfacer una necesidad documentada y de mantener la relación médico-paciente.

Por lo menos en cuanto a las cuestiones relacionadas con la población senescente, el sistema de salud de Estados Unidos está viendo las mismas

---

51. Amy Harmon, "A Soft Spot for Circuitry", [Un punto débil para los circuitos] *The New York Times*. 5 de julio de 2010, https://www.nytimes.com/2010/07/05/science/05robot.html?_r=2&pagewanted=1.

necesidades como las que se tratan con la IA en Japón. En Estados Unidos existe una creciente inquietud por la falta de apoyo suficiente para los pacientes de edad avanzada y esta preocupación se mencionó en un informe fechado en marzo de 2019 y publicado por la Administración de Donald Trump.[52] El informe Emerging Technologies to Support an Aging Population (Tecnologías emergentes para apoyar a una población senescente), indica claramente que el modelo de atención médica actual simplemente no está funcionando y que deben implementarse tecnologías emergentes para reducir la carga impuesta sobre los actuales proveedores de salud. Con la implementación de esta tecnología, Estados Unidos dependería menos de los auxiliares de la salud en el hogar, el cual es un campo en expansión debido al gran número de personas que requieren de este servicio. Sin embargo, es probable que cuestiones sobre los bajos salarios y las demandas físicas del trabajo continúen contribuyendo a la escasez de auxiliares de la salud en el hogar dentro de la fuerza laboral.[53] La falta de acceso a cuidados médicos por parte de la población de Estados Unidos no es, ciertamente, el único entorno donde las deficiencias documentadas en cuanto a la atención actual puedan ser o ya hayan sido subsanadas con la tecnología.

Las poblaciones rurales plantean un desafío particular para el modelo de atención médica moderno. Con sistemas hospitalarios más centralizados y concentrados en las ciudades más grandes del país, los médicos se han alejado aún más del ideal del médico de pueblo que podía hacer visitas a domicilio. Los desafíos planteados por los pacientes en áreas lejanas han dado pie a que la opción de la telemedicina sea más asequible.[54] Al implementar la capacidad de los pacientes para que vean a un médico de forma virtual, se evita que conduzcan al centro de salud más cercano, que busquen transporte cuando no se disponga de automóvil o que cuenten con que un médico vaya hasta donde se encuentren. Babylon Health se ha enfocado explícitamente en oportunidades para ayudar a estas poblaciones

---

52. Mark Mather, Paola Scommegna y Lillian Kilduff, "Fact Sheet: Aging in the United States" [Hoja de datos: envejecimiento en Estados Unidos], Population Reference Bureau, 15 de julio de 2019, https://www.prb.org/aging-unitedstates-fact-sheet/.

53. U.S. Bureau of Labor Statistics, "Home Health Aides and Personal Care Aides: Occupational Outlook Handbook," [Asistentes de salud en el hogar y asistentes de cuidado personal: manual de perspectivas ocupacionales] 4 de septiembre de 2019. https://www.bls.gov/ooh/healthcare/home-health-aides-and-personal-care-aides.htm.

54. Ahmed Hosney y Hugo J. W. L. Aerts, "Artificial Intelligence for Global Health" [Inteligencia artificial para la salud global]. American Association for the Advancement of Science, 22 de noviembre de 2019, https://science.sciencemag.org/content/366/6468/955.full.

lejanas. Después de aprobar el examen de licencia médica del Reino Unido, la IA de Babylon fue implementada en poblaciones apartadas de África, permitiendo que un sistema con muy pocos médicos atienda a un mayor número de pacientes y lo que es más importante, invertir más tiempo en aquellos pacientes que requieren mayor atención.[55] Babylon ha crecido desde entonces, con la compañía con sede en Londres que está desarrollando una aplicación para iOS y para Android destinada a poner esa misma atención médica de primera línea al alcance de cualquier persona en Estados Unidos que cuente con un teléfono inteligente. La idea detrás de la tecnología es simple: encontrar la forma de aumentar el acceso a la atención médica en un sistema donde dicho acceso sea un reto.

Si la IA como médico de primera línea puede interactuar con un paciente y diagnosticar enfermedades y padecimientos comunes como las alergias, el resfriado común e incluso la gripe, entonces la interacción humana médico-paciente puede, en teoría, reservarse para casos más complicados. Como el médico no tendría que destinar tiempo para atender a aquellos pacientes que pudieran ser diagnosticados de manera rápida y fácil con el uso de IA, podría entonces tener una conversación más larga y a fondo con pacientes que requieran de una atención más específica. Esto no solo mantendría una relación médico-paciente entre un humano y alguien que toma decisiones médicas de IA de primera línea, sino que también profundizaría la relación médico-paciente entre el paciente humano y el médico humano. Sin embargo, muchos han estado prontos para señalar un problema en un modelo donde la IA es quien toma la decisión final con respecto al diagnóstico médico, incluso para casos sencillos. Conocido como el problema de la caja negra, la preocupación consiste en que, si el diagnóstico de un paciente proviene de una IA, incluso si la decisión final parece tener sentido, no existe manera de que un ser humano entienda por qué se hizo ese diagnóstico.[56]

La naturaleza de la caja negra de la IA puede parecer frustrante debido a la incapacidad para comprender plenamente las razones por las que una IA tomó esa decisión, sin embargo, es probable que esta frustración tenga su origen en prácticas médicas anteriores con respecto a las relaciones

---

55. Babylon Health, "Babylon AI Achieves Equivalent Accuracy with Human Doctors." [La IA de Babylon logra una precisión equivalente a la de los médicos humanos]
56. Robin C. Feldman, Ehrik Aldana y Kara Stein. 2019. "Artificial Intelligence in the Health Care Space: How can we trust what we cannot know"[La inteligencia artificial en el ámbito del cuidado de la salud: ¿Cómo podemos confiar en lo que no podemos saber?, *Stanford Law & Policy Review* 30 (2): 406.

médico-paciente. El problema de la caja negra plantea una cuestión ética muy similar a la observada con el predominio de los enfoques paternalistas hacia la medicina. La IA toma una decisión y se espera que el paciente acepte esa decisión sin cuestionarla. Con el avance de la medicina, pudo observarse un mayor deseo de autonomía en cuanto a la toma de decisiones médicas, con el fin de que los pacientes del entorno de atención médica occidental tuvieran más control sobre su propio cuidado médico.[57] Sin embargo, es posible que las futuras tecnologías no tengan este mismo problema conforme mejore la IA. Puede ser que la IA tome la decisión, sin embargo, al identificar el problema de la caja negra ahora, es muy probable que los investigadores diseñen las futuras tecnologías de IA para que tengan la capacidad de explicar por qué se llegaron a ciertas conclusiones según los datos suministrados. Dicho avance constituiría una increíble transición de la inteligencia artificial débil a la fuerte y para revalorar los anteriores ejemplos de sistemas de diagnóstico y de los sistemas de IA que aprueban exámenes de licencia médica, cuyos pasos hacia estos avances ya están teniendo lugar.

Sin necesidad de analizar más a fondo el potencial del paternalismo dentro de la IA frente a los hábitos paternalistas restantes de los médicos humanos cuyo propósito es la benevolencia, existe un punto adicional que sugiere que la caja negra no debe considerarse como un defecto significativo de las tecnologías de IA. Sencillamente, si una IA no es capaz de explicar completamente a un paciente por qué se tomó una decisión, esto no difiere del todo de un especialista que intenta explicar a fondo su razonamiento a un paciente sin conocimiento médico. La mala comunicación y los malentendidos entre médicos y pacientes están bien documentados en la literatura académica, lo cual indica que aunque, teóricamente, un médico cuenta con los medios para explicar su decisión, no siempre lo hace con precisión.[58] Lo anterior indica, sin embargo, que sin importar si es un médico humano o una IA del futuro quien diagnostica directamente a un paciente, igual deben tomarse las medidas necesarias para evitar la mala comunicación y mantener la confianza entre el paciente y su prestador de servicios médicos. Con el desarrollo de sistemas de IA, los investigadores deben esforzarse por mitigar el problema de la caja negra. Sin embargo, su existencia hoy en día dentro de la IA, sin duda, no indica por sí solo que la tecnología no sea ética.

---

57. Beauchamp y Childress, *Principios*, 40.
58. Dennis Rosen. *Vital Conversations: Improving Communication Between Doctors and Patients* [Conversaciones vitales: mejora de la comunicación entre médicos y pacientes]. New York: Columbia University Press, 2014, 161–162.

Incluso en un futuro en el que el problema de la caja negra se supere o nosotros como sociedad confiemos plenamente en las decisiones de la IA sin ninguna explicación, todavía quedarán otros problemas realistas sobre el uso de la IA. Una de las inquietudes más palpables de las personas que se apoyan en la IA en vez de su propia experiencia, es la posibilidad de que una persona ignore su propia inteligencia y confíe en la tecnología, incluso cuando sea obvio que está equivocada. Un ejemplo de este fenómeno, ya observado con la IA, es el de las muchas personas que han seguido las indicaciones de un GPS directamente hacia alguna masa de agua.[59] Esas personas ignoraron su propio sentido de orientación, hicieron caso omiso de todas las señales que les indicaban que los caminos por los que conducían no eran aptos y siguieron las indicaciones de su GPS hasta verse al final, sumergidos en el agua. Si bien nadie resultó lesionado en estas situaciones y el resultado final es un automóvil dañado, un poco de vergüenza y un titular decente en el periódico local al día siguiente, no todos los casos de dependencia de la tecnología defectuosa son tan inermes. Al mencionar de nuevo a Watson for Oncology, finalmente quedó claro que los planes de tratamiento que proponía no eran efectivos para los pacientes y que pudieron haber causado más daño que beneficio. Si los médicos solo hubieran atendido las sugerencias de la IA en lugar de utilizar su propia experiencia médica para reconocer cuando algo no tenía sentido respecto al tratamiento del paciente, esto pudiera muy bien haber llevado a la muerte del mismo. Una muerte ocasionada directamente por la información inexacta que suministra una IA y la confianza de un médico de que la IA "sabía más".

El problema de la caja negra y la posibilidad de que un médico ignore su propia experiencia y se remita por completo a una IA implementada en un sistema de salud constituyen, ciertamente, cuestiones que deben ser abordadas conforme la IA se entrelaza aún más y de manera inevitable, en la toma de decisiones de corte médico. Sin embargo, estas inquietudes no deben obstaculizar la aplicación de futuras tecnologías en los sistemas de cuidado de la salud. Reconociendo que, en función de las tendencias actuales de las tecnologías de IA a nivel mundial y en Estados Unidos, es imperativo discutir las aplicaciones éticas de las tecnologías de un futuro cercano. Como se mencionó anteriormente, el siguiente paso lógico de

---

59. Malone Kircher. "Yet Another Person Listens to GPS App and Drives Car into Lake." [Una persona más sigue ciegamente el GPS y conduce el auto hacia el lago] *Intelligencer*, 24 de enero de 2018. https://nymag.com/intelligencer/2018/01/waze-app-directs-driver-to-drive-car-into-lake-champlain.html.

la IA con respecto a la atención médica es el de la IA como médico de primera línea. La clave para implementar éticamente dichos sistemas de IA dentro de un entorno médico tiene dos vertientes: la IA debe cubrir una necesidad dentro del entorno de atención médica y el paciente debe ser capaz de compenetrarse con la IA para poder mantener la relación médico-paciente. Puede haber determinados consultorios médicos o una cierta rama de un sistema hospitalario con distintas facetas de este criterio, pero existe un sistema de salud en Estados Unidos que, en conjunto, facilitaría las bases para la aplicación ética de los médicos de IA de primera línea: la Administración de Salud de los Veteranos (VHA, por sus siglas en inglés).

Para abordar la primera necesidad en el uso ético de IA como médico de primera línea, la VHA cuenta con un historial bien documentado de largos tiempos de espera, de atención inadecuada y de una reputación generalizada de no satisfacer las necesidades de sus pacientes. Incluso el proceso para recibir las prestaciones a través de la VHA puede ser una pesadilla para algunos miembros del servicio de las Fuerzas Armadas de Estados Unidos. Entre los ejemplos ciertamente desastrosos sobre el mal manejo de las peticiones por discapacidad de la VHA, un hombre que había sufrido lesiones documentadas durante su servicio en la Guardia Costera pasó treinta y cuatro años apelando ante el Departamento de Asuntos de los Veteranos para recibir las prestaciones por discapacidad.[60] Otra veterana con diabetes tuvo que batallar para recibir atención médica, finalmente perdió un pie y para cuando su solicitud fue aprobada, ya le habían amputado el otro pie.[61] Incluso cuando a un veterano se le otorga la aprobación para atenderse médicamente o recibir un pago, los problemas persisten.

La VHA cuenta con un historial de veteranos que no pueden programar citas oportunas, incluso en el caso de enfermedades inminentemente mortales.[62] Esta cuestión llegó a los titulares de Estados Unidos cuando la CNN publicó un informe sobre el sistema de salud de los Asuntos de los Veteranos en Phoenix, en el estado de Arizona, donde fallecieron algunos veteranos,

---

60. Dave Philipps, "Veterans Claiming Disability Pay Face Wall of Denial and Delays"[Veteranos que reclaman pago por discapacidad enfrentan una muralla de negaciones y demoras], *The New York Times*, 13 de noviembre de 2017, https://www.nytimes.com/2017/11/13/us/veterans-affairs-department-benefits-delays.html.
61. Dave Phillips, "Veterans Claiming Disability Pay."[Veteranos reclaman pago por discapacidad]
62. *Waiting for Care: Examining Patient Wait Times at VA Committee on Veterans 'Affairs Committee on Veterans' Affairs*, 2013, Declaración del Presidente Mike Coffman, Subcomité de Supervisión e Investigaciones de Asuntos de los Veteranos. http://search.ebscohost.com/login.aspx?direct=true&AuthType=ip,shib&db=cat07006a&AN=cwru.b4081068&site=eds-live.

debido a que nunca pudieron ser atendidos por un médico. La CNN expuso que dichas muertes habían sido el resultado de una "lista secreta" creada por los gerentes de la VHA para ocultar el hecho de que cerca de 1,500 pacientes se habían visto obligados a esperar durante meses para poder ver a un médico, lo que a la larga ocasionó la muerte de por lo menos cuarenta veteranos debido a la falta de atención médica.[63] La VHA ha tomado medidas para identificar áreas en las que los tiempos de espera exceden el requisito de que los pacientes sean atendidos de manera oportuna, pero surgen las dificultades al tratar de definir lo que es un largo tiempo de espera para los pacientes, así como la lucha con un sistema que programará una cita para un veterano pero que, a fin de cuentas, la reprogramará varias veces.[64] Ha habido avances desde el escándalo de Phoenix, pero los tiempos de espera siguen preocupando a la VHA, incluso con las medidas tomadas en los últimos años para mejorar los sistemas de programación e incrementar la supervisión.[65] En tanto que el acto de programar –y a menudo reprogramar– en sí, haya sido mencionado como una razón para explicar los largos tiempos de espera, otro problema es el de la falta de personal médico.

Las proyecciones sugieren que para el año 2025 habrá una escasez de médicos a nivel nacional en Estados Unidos, lo que afectará particularmente a los sistemas hospitalarios rurales y a aquellos que no tengan puedan ofrecer salarios competitivos.[66] Desafortunadamente, la VHA encaja con frecuencia en ambas categorías, lo que provoca una mayor preocupación por los VAMC (Centros Médicos de los Asuntos de los Veteranos) que no cuentan con suficientes fondos. Ya se han presentado problemas potenciales ocasionados por la futura escasez de médicos en la VHA. Entre el 2011 y el 2015, el número de médicos que abandonaron la VHA se incrementó cada

---

63. Scott Bronstein and Drew Griffin, "A Fatal Wait: Veterans Languish and Die on a VA Hospital's Secret List,"[Una espera fatal: los veteranos languidecen y mueren en la lista secreta de un hospital de VA] *CNN* (Cable News Network, 24 de abril de 2014), https://www.cnn.com/2014/04/23/health/veterans-dying-health-care-delays/index.html.

64. Brendan McGarry, "VA Audit Confirms Veterans 'Wait Times Complaints," [Auditoría a VA confirma quejas de tiempos de espera de los veteranos] *Military.com*, 2014, https://www.military.com/daily-news/2014/06/10/va-audit-confirms-veterans-wait-times-complaints.html.

65. Patricia Kime, "5 Years After Nationwide Scandal, VA Still Struggles to Track Wait Times," [Cinco años después del escándalo a nivel nacional, VA aún lucha por rastrear los tiempos de espera] *Military.com*, 26 de julio de 2019, https://www.military.com/daily-news/2019/07/26/5-years-after-nationwide-scandal-va-still-struggles-track-wait-times.html

66. Department of Health and Human Services, Health Resources and Services Administration, Designated Health Professional Shortage Areas Statistic, HRSA Data Warehouse, 2017.

año fiscal debido a las jubilaciones y a las renuncias voluntarias.[67] En el año 2018, un informe de la Oficina de Rendición de Cuentas del Gobierno de Estados Unidos (GAO, por sus siglas en inglés), mostró claramente que la VHA se esfuerza por reclutar y retener a médicos de tiempo completo en la VHA y, si bien se han tomado las medidas para incrementar dicha retención, muchos de los VAMC dependen de médicos de medio tiempo, de aquellos que trabajan como voluntarios o de médicos en formación que finalmente se van.[68] Es comprensible que la VHA haya identificado la contratación de nuevos médicos como una prioridad principal, pero en el año 2019, la GAO se dio cuenta que los intentos por aumentar el número de personal médico dieron como resultado, en efecto, más médicos, pero muchos de ellos carecían de las licencias necesarias para ejercer.[69] Un ejemplo particularmente indignante que figura en el informe es el de un médico a quien anteriormente se le había revocado su licencia debido a una negligencia hacia el paciente, había sido contratado por la VHA. Todos estos informes de los tiempos de espera de los pacientes, la disponibilidad de médicos y su contratación describen una clara imagen: la VHA necesita ayuda.

Si bien la IA no puede resolver todos los retos que enfrenta la VHA, la implementación de IA como médico de primera línea cubriría muchas de estos problemas arraigados al cumplir con el primero de los dos requisitos para que se implemente la IA de manera ética, como si fuera un médico de primera línea. Esta no sería la primera vez que la utilización de la IA de tal manera, fuera propuesta como una solución a la problemática de la VHA. En el año 2008, una audiencia ante la Comisión de Asuntos de los Veteranos presentó una propuesta para usar la IA para ampliar el sistema de procesamiento de reclamos de la VHA.[70] Como resultado de lo anteriormente comentado sobre el procesamiento de reclamos y del escándalo de la VHA de Phoenix, las propuestas presentadas en dicha audiencia no

67. *Steps Taken to Improve Physician Staffing, Recruitment, and Retention, but Challenges Remain* [Pasos tomados para mejorar la dotación de personal, el reclutamiento y la retención de médicos, pero los desafíos persisten]. Declaración de la directora de cuidados de la salud, Debra Draper ante el subcomité de salud, Committee on Veterans' Affairs, House of Representatives Veterans Health, 2018.
68. *Steps Taken to Improve Physician Staffing.*
69. Kathy Larin, "Veterans health administration: Greater focus on credentialing needed to prevent disqualified providers from delivering patient care," [VHA: se require de un mayor enfoque en cuanto a la acreditación para evitar que proveedores no calificados presten servicio a los pacientes] *Nova Science Publishers, Inc.* 2019: 205.
70. *The Use of Artificial Intelligence to Improve the U.S. Department of Veterans Affairs 'Claims Processing System,* 2008. Audiencia ante el Subcomité de Asistencia para Discapacitados y Asuntos Conmemorativos del Comité de Asuntos de los Veteranos de Guerra.

se tradujeron en muchas mejoras. Sin embargo, para el año 2021 está programada la implementación de un nuevo sistema de software que abarque toda la VHA con el propósito de mejorar en forma significativa los actuales procesos de programación y tiempos de espera.[71] Por supuesto que tomará tiempo ver si la adopción de la IA como software de programación de citas se traducirá en una reducción de las quejas presentadas con respecto a las dificultades que enfrentan los pacientes para poder ver a un médico de forma oportuna. Incluso si el sistema facilita darle seguimiento a la programación de citas y a agendarlas desde un principio, el problema de la falta de médicos calificados continuará y deberá ser solucionado. El uso actual de Watson for Oncology en los más de setenta centros VAMC tiene como propósito apoyar a los médicos, pero la futura implementación de la IA como si fuera un médico de primera línea, ayudaría directamente a mitigar la necesidad de mano de obra en general. Al utilizar la IA como si fuera un médico de primera línea, los pacientes de la VHA podrían de inmediato, programar una cita con una IA para recibir atención básica u obtener una referencia médica, aligerando la carga de los actuales médicos para que se dediquen a atender los problemas de los veteranos que requieran de una atención más minuciosa.

Al reconocer que el uso de la IA como si fuera un médico de primera línea cubriría muchas de las necesidades documentadas de la VHA, queda todavía el segundo requisito sobre el uso ético de dicha tecnología. Para poder utilizar éticamente este recurso, los miembros de las Fuerzas Armadas de Estados Unidos deben ser capaces de mantener la relación médico-paciente con una IA como médico de primera línea. Afortunadamente, durante su periodo de servicio, muchos miembros del servicio militar han demostrado la capacidad de conectarse a nivel personal con las tecnologías de vanguardia. Esto resulta evidente de manera específica con las unidades de eliminación de artefactos explosivos (EOD, por sus siglas en inglés) y en el uso de robots para la eliminación de bombas que tuvo su origen en el año 1972.[72] En los años que transcurrieron a partir de que estos robots se implementaran en el campo, las unidades de EOD han demostrado una asombrosa capacidad para forjar vínculos emocionales con el robot, a tal

---

71. Patricia Kime, "5 Years After Nationwide Scandal." [Cinco años después del escándalo a nivel nacional]

72. Military.com, "The Very First Bomb Disposal Robot" [El primer robot para la desactivación de armas], 15 de enero de 2014, https://www.military.com/video/ammunition-and-explosives/explosive-ordnance-disposal/the-first-bomb-disposal-robot/3059244734001.

grado, que las unidades inventan nombres para el robot y lo tratan como a una mascota.[73] Algunas unidades han desarrollado relaciones con sus robots lo suficientemente sólidas de manera que cuando el robot sufre daños irreparables, la unidad muestra un genuino dolor y lleva a cabo un funeral para su "compañero soldado".[74] Los ejemplos de las unidades de EOD y sus robots caídos demuestran que los soldados son capaces de entablar relaciones con entidades que no son humanas. Los veteranos con trastorno por estrés postraumático (TEPT, por sus siglas en inglés) también han mostrado la disposición de revelar más información con un chatbot de IA de la que harían en un habitual entorno médico.[75] Esta relación directa con la IA es probable que aumentar gracias a la evidente disposición de los militares de recurrir a la tecnología avanzada para satisfacer las necesidades de los miembros del servicio militar.

A lo largo de la historia, la investigación militar ha ido a la vanguardia de los avances médicos. Si bien la causa principal que originó la necesidad de desarrollar esa tecnología es a menudo trágica, el ejército siempre ha propiciado un entorno donde se ha visto un enorme avance de las extremidades protésicas al igual que han mejorado los métodos para recuperar las extremidades y aumentar su funcionalidad.[76] Incluso cosas tan aparentemente básicas como el torniquete o la producción en masa de antibióticos se originaron en un contexto militar.[77] Estos avances pasaron de un contexto militar a formar parte de todos los sistemas de salud y se espera que ocurra lo mismo con los avances médicos en el futuro.

La investigación desclasificada de la Agencia de Proyectos de Investigación Avanzada de la Defensa (DARPA, por sus siglas en inglés) en curso, muestra

---

73. Doree Armstrong, "Emotional Attachment to Robots Could Affect Outcome on Battlefield,"[El apego emocional a los robots podría afectar el resultado en el campo de batalla] Office of Minority Affairs Diversity, 13 de septiembre de 2013, https://www.washington.edu/news/2013/09/17/emotional-attachment-to-robots-could-affect-outcome-on-battlefield/.

74. Megan Garber, "Funerals for Fallen Robots"[Funerales para los robots caídos], The Atlantic. 20 de septiembre de 2013. https://www.theatlantic.com/technology/archive/2013/09/funerals-for-fallen-robots/279861/.

75. Myrthe L. Tielman et al., "A Therapy System for Post-Traumatic Stress Disorder." [Un sistema de terapia para el trastorno de estrés postraumático]

76. Melissa Block, "Orthotic Brace Takes Soldiers from Limping to Leaping" [Aparato ortopédico lleva a los soldados de cojear a saltar], NPR, 31 de marzo de 2014, https://www.npr.org/sections/health-shots/2014/03/31/295328707/orthotic-brace-takes-soldiers-from-limping-to-leaping.

77. Leah Samuel, "6 Battlefield Medical Innovations That Moved to Mainstream Medicine," [Seis innovaciones médicas en el campo de batalla que pasaron a formar parte de la medicina convencional] STAT, 10 de noviembre de 2017, https://www.statnews.com/2017/11/10/medical-innovations-war/.

interés por implementar tecnologías de IA médica en las Fuerzas Armadas de Estados Unidos. Uno de los programas de la DARPA, el Warfighter Analytics using Smartphones for Health (Análisis de la Salud de los Soldados mediante el uso de Teléfonos Inteligentes, o WASH, por sus siglas en inglés), tiene como objetivo la utilización de la tecnología integrada en un teléfono inteligente para poder monitorear la salud y la condición general de un soldado, hasta el punto de identificar cambios mínimos en el modo de andar de un soldado, su tensión muscular y su nivel de transpiración.[78] Otro proyecto anunciado en el año 2019, el Bioelectronics for Tissue Regeneration (Bioelectrónica para la Regeneración de Tejidos, o BETR, por sus siglas en inglés), tiene como objetivo la utilización de IA combinándola con sensores para monitorear la respuesta corporal ante estimulaciones bioquímicas o biofísicas al tejido con el fin de suministrar datos a solenoides que podrán tener la capacidad de curar heridas.[79] Conforme avance la tecnología militar y la IA se integre más con las interacciones dentro del ejército, mayor será el número de ejemplos de miembros del ejército que se conecten con la tecnología durante su periodo de servicio. Y además de las interacciones que los miembros de las Fuerzas Armadas de los Estados Unidos tengan con la IA durante su periodo de servicio, también tendrán acceso a la tecnología de IA desarrollada para el consumo en masa.

Estas interacciones con la IA crean entonces, la base sobre la cual los miembros del servicio que busquen tratamiento a través de la VHA puedan recibirlo de manera oportuna e incluso conservar de esta manera, la relación médico-paciente con la IA en su papel de médico de primera línea. Es comprensible que no todos los miembros del servicio tengan el mismo nivel de interacción con la IA, sobre todo aquellos pacientes de edad avanzada que no interactuaron con la IA durante su periodo de servicio. Con el fin de apegarse mejor al uso ético de la IA como médico de primera línea, los miembros del servicio que busquen tratamiento en un VAMC deben tener la opción de primero interactuar, ya sea con una IA, o de esperar hasta que un médico humano pueda atenderlos. Hacer lo contrario, pedirle a una persona que no estaría dispuesta a hablar con un chatbot o a ser atendida por una IA para un diagnóstico de un resfriado o una gripe y que, a pesar de sentirse

---

78. Jonathan M. Smith, "Warfighter Analytics Using Smartphones for Health (WASH)" [Análisis de la salud de los soldados mediante el uso de teléfonosiInteligentes]. https://www.darpa.mil/program/warfighter-analytics-using-smartphones-for-health.
79. Dr. Paul Sheehan, "Bioelectronics for Tissue Regeneration (BETR)" [Bioelectrónica para la regeneración de tejidos o BERT]. https://www.darpa.mil/program/bioelectronics-for-tissue-regeneration.

incómoda, lo haga, menoscabaría la relación médico-paciente y desvirtuaría la implementación de la tecnología como poco ética. Sin embargo, debido a la naturaleza de la progresiva relación de la humanidad con la IA en general y a los indicativos de futuras aplicaciones dentro de las Fuerzas Armadas de Estados Unidos, es probable que en los próximos años se aprecie un incremento en el número de pacientes dispuestos a interactuar con una IA como primera instancia. Como se discutió anteriormente en relación con los pacientes con TEPT, sus interacciones con un chatbot y el éxito en general de las citas de telesalud que están fácilmente disponibles, puede ser que los pacientes prefieran hablar con una IA si eso significa que pueden ser atendidos en ese momento.

En el corazón de la implementación de la IA en la medicina está el deseo de brindar una mejor atención, más precisa y accesible. En muchos sentidos, proponer la aplicación de la IA como un médico de primera línea en un sistema de salud de Estados Unidos plantea un mayor desafío debido la arraigada desconfianza social en perjuicio de la IA. Las cuestiones éticas que se basan en esta desconfianza no han podido, no obstante, detener los avances tecnológicos y ahora es imperativo darle un giro al diálogo de "¿debe permitirse la IA?" a "¿cómo debe implementarse la IA?" Para garantizar el uso ético de las futuras tecnologías en un sistema de salud, deben cumplirse dos requisitos: la tecnología debe satisfacer una necesidad documentada y la implementación de la tecnología no debe dañar el potencial para el desarrollo de la relación médico-paciente.

La incapacidad documentada de la Administración de Salud de los Veteranos (VHA) para atender plenamente a sus pacientes conforme al estándar establecido, podría replantearse mediante el uso de la IA como médico de primera línea. No solo eso, sino que muchos miembros de las Fuerzas Armadas de Estados Unidos que en el futuro busquen atenderse en los VAMC, ya habrán interactuado y desarrollado una relación única con las tecnologías de IA durante su periodo de servicio. Estas interacciones les daría mayor capacidad de mantener la confianza en una decisión médica cuando la IA sea el médico, conservando la relación médico-paciente. Es posible que la IA no pueda del todo, desempeñarse todavía como un médico de primera línea, pero en este momento es indispensable identificar la forma de implementarla éticamente en el futuro. Si bien las futuras tecnologías de la IA contribuirán sin duda a mejorar la atención médica en general, la Administración de Salud de Veteranos apuesta a beneficiarse enormemente de esta tecnología y proporciona un entorno en el que la implementación de la IA pueda apegarse a los principios base de la ética médica occidental.

Referencias

American Hospital Association. "Fact Sheet: Telehealth." February 2019. https://www.aha.org/system/files/2019-02/fact-sheet-telehealth-2-4-19.pdf.

Ana, Cat. "Why the Japanese Find Deep Love with Deep Learning." *Medium. Becoming Human: Artificial Intelligence Magazine*, February 12, 2019. https://becominghuman.ai/why-the-japanese-find-deep-love-with-deep-learning-829e1bb629c2.

Armstrong, Doree. "Emotional Attachment to Robots Could Affect Outcome on Battlefield." Office of Minority Affairs Diversity. September 13, 2013. https://www.washington.edu/news/2013/09/17/emotional-attachment-to-robots-could-affect-outcome-on-battlefield/.

Asimov, Isaac. "Runaround" *I, Robot*. Greenwich, CT: Fawcett Publications, 1950.

Bickmore, Timothy W., Suzanne E. Mitchell, Brian W. Jack, Michael K. Paasche-Orlow, Laura M. Pfeifer, and Julie O'Donnell. "Response to a Relational Agent by Hospital Patients with Depressive Symptoms." *Interacting with Computers* 22, no. 4 (2010): 289–98.

Block, Melissa. "Orthotic Brace Takes Soldiers from Limping to Leaping." *NPR*, March 31, 2014. https://www.npr.org/sections/health-shots/2014/03/31/295328707/orthotic-brace-takes-soldiers-from-limping-to-leaping.

Bronstein, Scott, and Drew Griffin. "A Fatal Wait: Veterans Languish and Die on a VA Hospital's Secret List." *CNN*. Cable News Network, April 24, 2014. https://www.cnn.com/2014/04/23/health/veterans-dying-health-care-delays/index.html.

Builddie. "The Role of Artificial Intelligence in Wildlife Conservation." *Medium*. May 15, 2019. https://medium.com/builddie/the-role-of-artificial-intelligence-in-wildlife-conservation-5dc3af2b4222.

Business Wire. "Pacificor Names Latham & Watkins to Field Terminator Inquiries." Berkshire Hathaway. February 17, 2010. http://www.businesswire.com/news/home/20100217005514/en/Pacificor-Names-Latham-Watkins-Field-Terminator-Inquiries.

Eakins, Christopher, Wendy D. Ellis, Sumit Pruthi, David P. Johnson, Marta Hernanz-Schulman, Chang Yu, and J. Herman Kan. "Second Opinion Interpretations by Specialty Radiologists at a Pediatric Hospital: Rate of Disagreement and Clinical Implications." *American Journal of Roentgenology* 199, no. 4 (2012): 916–20.

Babylon Health, "Babylon AI Achieves Equivalent Accuracy with Human Doctors in Global Healthcare First." PR Newswire: News Distribution, Targeting and Monitoring. June 27, 2018. https://www.prnewswire.com/news-releases/babylon-ai-achieves-equivalent-accuracy-with-human-doctors-in-global-health-care-first-686718631.html.

Beauchamp, Thomas L., and James F. Childress. *Principles of Biomedical Ethics*. New York: Oxford University Press, 2013

Berner, Eta S. and Tonya J. La Lande, "Overview of Clinical Decision Support Systems," in *Clinical Decision Support Systems: Theory and Practice,* ed. Eta S. Berner. Switzerland: Springer International Press, 2016.

Bresnick, Jennifer. "Artificial Intelligence in Healthcare Market to See 40% CAGR Surge." HealthITAnalytics, July 24, 2017. https://healthitanalytics.com/news/artificial-intelligence-in-healthcare-market-to-see-40-cagr-surge.

Brown, Eric. "Watson: The *Jeopardy!* Challenge and beyond." 2013 IEEE 12th International Conference on Cognitive Informatics and Cognitive Computing, 2013.

Brynjolfsson, Erik, and Andrew McAfee. The Second Machine Age: Work, Progress, and Prosperity in a Time of Brilliant Technologies. Vancouver, BC: Langara College, 2018.

"Cleveland Clinic Express Care® Online." Cleveland Clinic. Accessed April 29, 2019. https://my.clevelandclinic.org/online-services/express-care-online.

Dyce, Andrew. "Our 10 Favorite Killer A.I.'s in Movies." Screen Rant, April 18, 2014. https://screenrant.com/artificial-intelligence-movies-evil-computers/.

Ehrenkranz, Melanie. "Facial Recognition Flags Woman on Bus Ad for 'Jaywalking' in China." Gizmodo. November 26, 2018. https://gizmodo.com/facial-recognition-flags-woman-on-bus-ad-for-jaywalking-1830654750.

Feldman, Robin C., Ehrik Aldana, and Kara Stein. 2019. "Artificial Intelligence in the Health Care Space: How can we trust what we cannot know." *Stanford Law & Policy Review* 30 (2): 399–419.

Garber, Megan. "Funerals for Fallen Robots." *The Atlantic.* September 20, 2013. https://www.theatlantic.com/technology/archive/2013/09/funerals-for-fallen-robots/279861/.

Hall, Mark A., Elizabeth Dugan, Beiyao Zheng, and Aneil K. Mishra. "Trust in Physicians and Medical Institutions: What Is It, Can It Be Measured, and Does It Matter?" *The Milbank Quarterly* 79, no. 4 (2001): 613–39.

Harmon, Amy. "A Soft Spot for Circuitry." *The New York Times.* July 5, 2010. https://www.nytimes.com/2010/07/05/science/05robot.html?_r=2&pagewanted=1.

Hosny, Ahmed, and Hugo J. W. L. Aerts. "Artificial Intelligence for Global Health." *American Association for the Advancement of Science*, November 22, 2019. https://science.sciencemag.org/content/366/6468/955.full.

Heckerman, David E., and Edward H. Shortliffe. "From Certainty Factors to Belief Networks." *Artificial Intelligence in Medicine* 4, no. 1 (1992): 35–52.

Iannitti, Tommaso, Alessandro Di Cerbo, Julio Cesar Morales-Medina, and Beniamino Palmieri. "Narrative Review of Telemedicine Consultation in Medical Practice." Patient Preference and Adherence, 2015, 65.

IBM. "Watson Overview." The DeepQA Research Team, July 25, 2016. https://researcher.watson.ibm.com/researcher/view_group.php?id=2099.

IBM Newsroom. "Manipal Hospitals Announces National Launch of IBM Watson for Oncology" IBM, July 26, 2016. https://www-03.ibm.com/press/in/en/pressrelease/50290.wss.

Ito, Joi. "Why Westerners Fear Robots and the Japanese Do Not." Wired. Conde Nast, July 30, 2018. https://www.wired.com/story/ideas-joi-ito-robot-overlords/.

Karches, Kyle E. 2018. "Against the IDoctor: Why Artificial Intelligence Should Not Replace Physician Judgment." *Theoretical Medicine and Bioethics* 39 (2): 91–110.

Kircher, Malone. "Yet Another Person Listens to GPS App and Drives Car Into Lake." *Intelligencer*, January 24, 2018. https://nymag.com/intelligencer/2018/01/waze-app-directs-driver-to-drive-car-into-lake-champlain.html.

Kime, Patricia. "5 Years After Nationwide Scandal, VA Still Struggles to Track Wait Times." Military.com, July 26, 2019. https://www.military.com/daily-news/2019/07/26/5-years-after-nationwide-scandal-va-still-struggles-track-wait-times.html.

Krupinski, Elizabeth A., Kevin S. Berbaum, Robert T. Caldwell, Kevin M. Schartz, and John Kim. "Long Radiology Workdays Reduce Detection and Accommodation Accuracy." *Journal of the American College of Radiology* 7, no. 9 (2010): 698–704.

Larin, Kathy. "Veterans health administration: Greater focus on credentialing needed to prevent disqualified providers from delivering patient care." Nova Science Publishers, Inc. 2019: 205-284.

Lee, Don. "Desperate for Workers, Aging Japan Turns to Robots for Healthcare." Los Angeles Times. July 25, 2019. https://www.latimes.com/world-nation/story/2019-07-25/desperate-for-workers-aging-japan-turns-to-robots-for-healthcare.

Matchar, Emily. "AI Plant and Animal Identification Helps Us All Be Citizen Scientists." Smithsonian.com. Smithsonian Institution, June 7, 2017. https://www.smithsonianmag.com/innovation/ai-plant-and-animal-identification-helps-us-all-be-citizen-scientists-180963525/.

Mather, Mark, Paola Scommegna, and Lillian Kilduff. "Fact Sheet: Aging in the United States." Population Reference Bureau, July 15, 2019. https://www.prb.org/aging-unitedstates-fact-sheet/

McGarry, Brendan. "VA Audit Confirms Veterans' Wait Times Complaints." Military.com, 2014. https://www.military.com/daily-news/2014/06/10/va-audit-confirms-veterans-wait-times-complaints.html.

Military.com. "The Very First Bomb Disposal Robot." January 15, 2014. https://www.military.com/video/ammunition-and-explosives/explosive-ordnance-disposal/the-first-bomb-disposal-robot/3059244734001.

National Science and Technology Council. "Emerging Technologies to Support an Aging Population." March 2019. https://www.whitehouse.gov/wp-content/uploads/2019/03/Emerging-Tech-to-Support-Aging-2019.pdf.

Oxford English Dictionary Online. "Artificial Intelligence." November 2019. Oxford: Oxford University Press. https://www.oed.com/view/Entry/271625?redirectedFrom=artificial+intelligence#eid.

Philipps, Dave. "Veterans Claiming Disability Pay Face Wall of Denials and Delays." *The New York Times.* November 13, 2017. https://www.nytimes.com/2017/11/13/us/veterans-affairs-department-benefits-delays.html.

Polakovic, Gary. "The next Big Effort in AI: Keeping L.A.'s Water Flowing Post-Earthquake." USC News, October 4, 2019. https://news.usc.edu/160680/ai-la-water-supply-earthquake-usc-research/.

Ross, Casey, and Ike Swetlitz. "IBM's Watson supercomputer recommended 'unsafe and incorrect' cancer treatments, internal documents show." *STAT,* July 25, 2018. https://www.statnews.com/2018/07/25/ibm-watson-recommended-unsafe-incorrect-treatments/.

Rosen, Dennis. *Vital Conversations: Improving Communication Between Doctors and Patients.* New York: Columbia University Press, 2014.

Russell, Stuart J., and Peter Norvig. *Artificial Intelligence a Modern Approach.* Boston: Pearson, 2016.

Samuel, Leah. "6 Battlefield Medical Innovations That Moved to Mainstream Medicine." *STAT*, November 10, 2017. https://www.statnews.com/2017/11/10/medical-innovations-war/.

Si, Ma, and Cheng Yu. "Chinese Robot Becomes World's First Machine to Pass Medical Exam." November 10, 2017. http://www.chinadaily.com.cn/bizchina/tech/2017-11/10/content_34362656.htm.

Sheehan, Dr. Paul. "Bioelectronics for Tissue Regeneration (BETR)." https://www.darpa.mil/program/bioelectronics-for-tissue-regeneration.

Smith, Jonathan M. "Warfighter Analytics Using Smartphones for Health (WASH)." https://www.darpa.mil/program/warfighter-analytics-using-smartphones-for-health.

Spitzer, Julie. "IBM's Watson recommended 'unsafe and incorrect' cancer treatments, STAT report finds." *Becker's Healthcare*, July 25, 2018. https://www.beckershospitalreview.com/artificial-intelligence/ibm-s-watson-recommended-unsafe-and-incorrect-cancer-treatments-stat-report-finds.html..

Strickland, Eliza. "How IBM Watson Overpromised and Underdelivered on AI Health Care." *IEEE Spectrum: Technology, Engineering, and Science News*. April 2, 2019. https://spectrum.ieee.org/biomedical/diagnostics/how-ibm-watson-overpromised-and-underdelivered-on-ai-health-care.

Tajitsu, Naomi. "Japanese Automakers Look to Robots to Aid the Elderly." *Scientific American*. April 12, 2017. https://www.scientificamerican.com/article/japanese-automakers-look-to-robots-to-aid-the-elderly/.

Tielman, Myrthe L., Mark A. Neerincx, Rafael Bidarra, Ben Kybartas, and Willem-Paul Brinkman. "A Therapy System for Post-Traumatic Stress Disorder Using a Virtual Agent and Virtual Storytelling to Reconstruct Traumatic Memories." *Journal of Medical Systems* 41, no. 8 (2017): 125.

Truschel, Jessica. "Top 25 Mental Health Apps for 2020: An Alternative to Therapy?" Psycom.net–Mental Health Treatment Resource Since 1986, March 19, 2020. https://www.psycom.net/25-best-mental-health-apps.

United States Bureau of Labor Statistics. "Home Health Aides and Personal Care Aides: Occupational Outlook Handbook," September 4, 2019. https://www.bls.gov/ooh/healthcare/home-health-aides-and-personal-care-aides.htm.

Vaidyam, Aditya, and John Torous. "Chatbots: What Are They and Why Care?" *Psychiatric Times*. June 27, 2019. https://www.psychiatrictimes.com/telepsychiatry/chatbots-what-are-they-and-why-care.

Vincent, James. "Twitter Taught Microsoft's Friendly AI Chatbot to Be a Racist Asshole in Less Than a Day." *The Verge*. March 24, 2016. https://www.theverge.com/2016/3/24/11297050/tay-microsoft-chatbot-racist.

Vincent, James. "Google's AI Thinks This Turtle Looks like a Gun, Which Is a Problem." *The Verge*. November 2, 2017. https://www.theverge.com/2017/11/2/16597276/google-ai-image-attacks-adversarial-turtle-rifle-3d-printed.

Yan, Alice. "How a Robot Passed China's Medical Licensing Exam." *South China Morning Post*, November 20, 2017. Accessed April 20, 2019.

Yu, V. L. "Antimicrobial Selection by a Computer. A Blinded Evaluation by Infectious Diseases Experts." *JAMA: The Journal of the American Medical Association* 242, no. 12 (1979): 1279–282.

L'intelligence artificielle en tant que clinicien : argument en faveur d'un recours éthique aux technologies futures dans le milieu médical

Sara Gaines

Aujourd'hui la science-fiction est devenue réalité. Dans le monde entier la présence de l'intelligence artificielle (IA) dans les sociétés humaines voit son influence s'accroître, des appareils de poche aux logiciels internationalisés. Un domaine en particulier, la médecine, se tient au fait des différentes applications de ces technologies aujourd'hui et à l'avenir. Il n'est donc pas surprenant que les outils technologiques de l'IA soient en passe d'être adoptés dans le domaine de la santé et que cette tendance s'accompagne d'une inquiétude grandissante au sujet des problèmes éthiques qui entourent leur mise en service. À mesure des avancées technologiques, des préoccupations éthiques ont toujours été présentes. Toutefois, un domaine en particulier devra figurer au centre des conversations à venir, la relation patient-médecin, car le développement et les applications des nouvelles technologies pourraient placer l'IA au centre de décisions médicales, venant donc potentiellement influencer cette relation. Une version de cette technologie que je qualifie volontiers d'intelligence artificielle clinicienne de première ligne de soin peut être adoptée de façon éthique en suivant deux critères. En premier lieu, ses outils technologiques devraient être employés dans des environnements où le recours à l'intelligence artificielle soulage l'engorgement du système hospitalier permettant ainsi un meilleur accès aux soins de santé. Deuxièmement, ces technologies devraient être adoptées dans des environnements où les patients ont démontré une capacité à établir une relation personnelle avec l'intelligence artificielle. Aux États-Unis un organisme hospitalier, la Veteran Health Administration, serait à même de mettre à profit l'intelligence artificielle clinicienne de première ligne de soin en adhérant à ces critères relationnels.

Il semble difficile de ne pas considérer les futures applications de l'IA en médecine étant donné qu'elle est déjà pleinement adoptée dans la société.

Le dictionnaire unilingue Oxford English Dictionary définit l'intelligence artificielle comme « la théorie et le développement de systèmes informatiques capables d'opérer des tâches requérant ordinairement le recours à l'intelligence humaine. »[1] Si on s'en tient à cette définition, de nombreuses technologies employées quotidiennement par les usagers de portables montrent combien l'IA est devenue indispensable dans la vie des gens dans le monde. Le téléphone qu'on a dans sa poche est capable de chercher rapidement le restaurant le mieux noté dans un rayon géographique réduit, ainsi que de fournir des indications pour vous y rendre. Tout un chacun a déjà fait l'expérience de voir sa recherche en ligne d'un objet donné se muer en publicités diverses pour le produit en question sur de nombreuses plateformes de réseaux sociaux et sites Web pourtant sans peu de lien avec la recherche initiale. Il est plus facile que jamais de trouver de nouveaux morceaux de musique grâce à des services de streaming faisant chaque jour de nouvelles suggestions d'écoute. Ce ne sont là que quelques exemples d'intelligence artificielle s'étant facilement intégrés à la vie quotidienne, la présence de l'IA continuant de s'imposer avec de nouvelles évolutions technologiques. Cependant, afin d'évaluer l'impact de l'intégration des nouveaux outils technologiques non seulement dans nos activités quotidiennes mais tout spécifiquement dans le milieu médical, il est impératif d'éclaircir la définition de l'IA proposée dans le dictionnaire.

L'IA distingue les tâches accomplies par l'humain de celles qui le sont par une technologie « capable d'opérer des tâches requérant ordinairement le recours à l'intelligence humaine » par les termes respectifs d'intelligence artificielle forte ou d'intelligence artificielle faible. Les technologies de l'IA faible relèvent de celles qui sont structurées autour des habilités humaines.[2] Il s'agit par exemple de raisonnements en termes de probabilités et de capacités de perception visuelle. D'autre part, l'IA forte englobe les technologies hypothétiques considérées comme équivalentes à l'intelligence humaine, ou même superhumaine, en termes de capacité à l'exécution de tâches intelligentes.[3] Les technologies basées sur l'IA forte pourraient appréhender le

---

1. Oxford English Dictionary Online, "artificial intelligence," November 2019. Oxford: Oxford University Press. https://www.oed.com/view/Entry/271625?redirectedFrom=artificial+intelligence#eid.
2. Stuart J. Russell and Peter Norvig, *Artificial Intelligence a Modern Approach* (Boston: Pearson, 2016)
3. Erik Brynjolfsson and Andrew McAfee, *The Second Machine Age: Work, Progress, and Prosperity in a Time of Brilliant Technologies* (Vancouver, BC: Langara College, 2018).

symbolisme, évoluer dans divers contextes sociaux, concevoir leurs propres mécanismes de pensée idéologique. Sous de nombreux aspects, cela reflète la distinction entre les technologies connues (faibles) et les technologies futures (fortes). En revanche, cette distinction n'est pas binaire, car elle évolue sur une échelle de gradation. De nombreuses technologies repoussent les limites des algorithmes de recherche ou des programmes conçus pour trouver la chanson suivante dans votre liste de lecture en se dirigeant vers ce qui fut un temps considéré comme de la science-fiction, et en fait encore partie à plus d'un titre. Dans la société, la perception de l'IA est influencée par la science-fiction qui convoque un grand nombre d'idées anciennes et nouvelles, dont certaines font appel aux technologies fondées sur l'IA forte et sur leur représentation. Ainsi, l'image qu'on se fait de l'IA à travers ces exemples fictifs peut tout aussi bien nuire ou contribuer à la manière dont les humains interagissent avec les innovations technologiques émergentes.

Quoique cela ne s'inscrive pas dans un phénomène global, les États-Unis font preuve d'une certaine défiance envers l'IA. L'IA théorique capable de pensée indépendante a souvent été dépeinte comme douteuse dans la culture américaine. Les peurs suscitées par l'IA furent d'ailleurs répertoriées dans le monde occidental bien avant que le citoyen lambda eût commencé à interagir avec l'IA au quotidien. En 1950, Isaac Asimov publia *Les Robots*, recueil de nouvelles traitant de robots équipés d'intelligence artificielle et de leurs interactions avec le monde autour d'eux. On peut trouver dans ces nouvelles les trois fameuses lois de la robotique :

1. Un robot ne peut porter atteinte à un être humain ni, restant passif, permettre qu'un être humain soit exposé au danger.
2. Un robot doit obéir aux ordres que lui donne un être humain, sauf si de tels ordres entrent en conflit avec la Première loi.
3. Un robot doit protéger son existence tant que cette protection n'entre pas en conflit avec la Première ou la Deuxième loi.[4]

Ces lois, revues et adaptées par de nombreux auteurs, dont Asimov lui-même, ont eu une grande influence sur la science-fiction et dans le domaine de l'éthique de l'intelligence artificielle durant des décennies. La plupart des ouvrages de fiction qui examinent les avancées de l'IA sont fondés sur l'extrapolation de situations résultant d'un désir de pousser ces lois à l'extrême ou encore d'aller à leur encontre, alors que l'IA devenue

---

4. Isaac Asimov, "Runaround" *I, Robot*. Greenwich, CT: Fawcett Publications, 1950. Traduction en français de Pierre Billon, "Cycle fermé", *Le Livre des robots*. Paris: Opta/Club du livre d'anticipation, 1967.

ennemie de l'humanité était supposée être à son service. Fondamentalement, une grande partie de la culture fondée sur l'IA aux États-Unis est une culture de la peur.

Un des exemples les plus emblématiques de cette peur apparaît dans la franchise Terminator dans laquelle l'intrigue est fondée sur la défaite de Skynet, une super-intelligence artificielle dotée d'une conscience (le point le plus élevé sur l'échelle de l'IA forte). L'année 1984 vit la sortie du premier d'une série de six films, et en 2010, la franchise composée de longs métrages, séries, jeux vidéo, bandes dessinées, manèges à thème ainsi que d'une pléthore de produits dérivés avait amassé plus de trois milliards de dollars de revenus bruts.[5] Deux films supplémentaires sont sortis depuis dans la même franchise. Pour la population américaine l'idée même de l'IA a quelque chose d'irrésistible ; dans ce cas précis, c'est le maléfique Skynet. À savoir que la franchise de Terminator n'est pas la seule qui ait réussi à fédérer un grand nombre de fans. Centré sur l'histoire d'une société humaine soumise à une IA pervertie, *The Matrix* constitue une autre franchise incontournable dans la culture populaire américaine avec un budget à hauteur de multimilliards de dollars. D'innombrables films, séries et ouvrages présentant des systèmes d'IA dévoyés sont sortis par la suite. Le trope a acquis une telle célébrité dans les médias aux États-Unis que des listes d'IA tueuses, connues comme les "killer AIs", peuvent contenir des ouvrages allant de la science-fiction pure et dure jusqu'à des dessins animés pour enfants.[6]

En revanche, le reste du monde ne partage pas cette vision de l'IA. En effet, la perception japonaise des technologies fondées sur l'IA est presque diamétralement opposée à la peur qu'elle suscite dans la culture populaire américaine. Les médias japonais représentent les robots et les technologies fondées sur l'IA forte comme des alliés, et dans de nombreux cas, comme des amants.[7] Une telle approche de l'IA peut être attribuée à des différences culturelles émanant de différents cadres de pensée religieuse présents au

---

5. Business Wire, "Pacificor Names Latham & Watkins to Field Terminator Inquiries," *Berkshire Hathaway*, February 17, 2010. https://web.archive.org/web/20170306034914/http://www.businesswire.com/news/home/20100217005514/en/Pacificor-Names-Latham-Watkins-Field-Terminator-Inquiries.
6. Andrew Dyce, "Our 10 Favorite Killer A.I.'s in Movies," *Screen Rant*, April 18, 2014. https://screenrant.com/artificial-intelligence-movies-evil-computers/.
7. Cat Ana, "Why the Japanese Find Deep Love with Deep Learning," *Medium* (*Becoming Human: Artificial Intelligence Magazine*, February 12, 2019), https://becominghuman.ai/why-the-japanese-find-deep-love-with-deep-learning-829e1bb629c2.

Japon.[8] L'histoire du bouddhisme et du Shintoïsme a conduit la société japonaise à considérer toutes les choses, qu'elles soient douées de raison ou non, comme étant dignes de respect, ce qui entre en contraste avec les notions judéo-chrétiennes de la suprématie de l'être humain au sommet de tout autre règne, si ce n'est celui de Dieu.[9] À travers sa capacité de voir de la vie en toute chose, la société japonaise devait être capable de l'envisager également dans l'IA et dans la robotique, ce qui l'amena nécessairement à percevoir ses objets technologiques comme les allié(e)s ou les amant(e)s dépeint(e)s dans ses médias. Même dans les conversations au sujet des outils technologiques à usage médical fondés sur l'IA, la volonté d'accepter un objet de cet ordre peut être directement attribuée au dessin animé des années 1950 intitulé Astro Boy.[10]

À l'opposé du visage amical attribué à l'IA au Japon, les avertissements contre l'IA dans la culture populaire américaine ne sont guère subtils. En effet, les films de ces franchises sont marqués par un sentiment d'inéluctabilité portant sur l'idée qu'un jour la science pourrait aller trop loin et que l'IA, censée être un atout pour l'humanité, pourrait soudain se retourner contre elle, nonobstant la présence des trois lois dans son code ou la prise de mesure de sécurité comme garde-fou. Il n'est pas étonnant que la recherche associant les termes « intelligence artificielle » et « trop loin » dans les pages Web des pays industrialisés puisse recueillir plus de 39.000 résultats.[11] En revanche, dans la réalité, ces craintes avérées n'ont pas mis fin aux progrès des technologies fondées sur l'IA. Ces développements n'ont pas toujours été couronnés de succès, quoique chaque avancée infructueuse ait planté les jalons de succès futurs.

Dans sa tentative d'inventer une IA qui soit assimilable à la présence humaine sur les réseaux sociaux, l'entreprise Microsoft s'est vite rendu compte que son robot social n'était pas à la hauteur de ces ambitions. En effet, le robot social Tay, dont le fonctionnement était fondé sur l'IA, fut doté de son propre compte sur Twitter en 2016, mais cette expérience peu concluante devait prendre fin au bout de seize heures de temps qui avaient été suffisantes pour voir Tay le chatbot poli et aimable se mettre

---

8. Joi Ito, "Why Westerners Fear Robots and the Japanese Do Not," *Wired* (Conde Nast, July 30, 2018), https://www.wired.com/story/ideas-joi-ito-robot-overlords/.

9. Joi Ito, "Why Westerners."

10. Don Lee, "Desperate for Workers, Aging Japan Turns to Robots for Healthcare," *Los Angeles Times*, July 25, 2019, https://www.latimes.com/world-nation/story/2019-07-25/desperate-for-workers-aging-japan-turns-to-robots-for-healthcare..

11. Results from a Google Scholar search on April 11, 2020, excluding patents and citations.

à proférer des insultes racistes.[12] De même, le logiciel de reconnaissance faciale employé par de nombreux utilisateurs sur leur téléphone portable a aussi démontré que l'IA est moins fiable lorsqu'elle est mise en service à grande échelle. Par exemple, la Chine a récemment mené une expérience de sécurité routière à grande échelle consistant à verbaliser les piétons qui traversent la rue en dehors des passages protégés : cette dernière s'est soldée en un nombre record de contraventions adressées à des acteurs et à des mannequins dont le visage était placardé sur les transports publics.[13] En outre, lorsqu'il ne s'agit pas de reconnaissance faciale mais de la reconnaissance d'objets, certains outils d'identification non spécialisés n'ont également pas eu le succès escompté. Par exemple, l'un d'entre eux prit une tortue pour une arme à feu.[14] Cependant, pour tout échec avéré, un jalon est posé en vertu du progrès.

Ces dernières années, des technologies fondées sur l'IA semblant être tout droit sorties d'un film de science-fiction et se rapprochant d'exemples d'IA forte ont rencontré un franc succès. L'IA de Google a certes pris une tortue pour un révolver, mais il y a par ailleurs de nombreuses applications spécialisées en reconnaissance d'objets permettant à leurs utilisateurs d'identifier un animal ou une plante rare dans son écosystème.[15] Les animaux présents dans les jardins ne sont pas les seuls à avoir été impactés par les avancées de l'IA ; on pense en cela aux drones équipés de technologies fondées sur l'IA mis en service pour mettre fin au braconnage en Afrique.[16] Dans le contexte urbain, on se tourne également vers l'IA pour résoudre des problèmes existants. La ville de Los Angeles s'en est remise à l'IA en tant que source de solutions potentielles pour gérer son réseau de canalisa-

---

12. James Vincent, "Twitter Taught Microsoft's Friendly AI Chatbot to Be a Racist Asshole in Less Than a Day." *The Verge*. March 24, 2016. https://www.theverge.com/2016/3/24/11297050/tay-microsoft-chatbot-racist.

13. Melanie Ehrenkranz, "Facial Recognition Flags Woman on Bus Ad for 'Jaywalking' in China." *Gizmodo*. November 26, 2018. https://gizmodo.com/facial-recognition-flags-woman-on-bus-ad-for-jaywalking-1830654750.

14. James Vincent, Google's AI Thinks This Turtle Looks like a Gun, Which Is a Problem." *The Verge*. November 2, 2017. https://www.theverge.com/2017/11/2/16597276/google-ai-image-attacks-adversarial-turtle-rifle-3d-printed.

15. Emily Matchar, "AI Plant and Animal Identification Helps Us All Be Citizen Scientists," Smithsonian.com (Smithsonian Institution, June 7, 2017), https://www.smithsonianmag.com/innovation/ai-plant-and-animal-identification-helps-us-all-be-citizen-scientists-180963525/.

16. Builddie, "The Role of Artificial Intelligence in Wildlife Conservation," *Medium*, May 15, 2019, https://medium.com/builddie/the-role-of-artificial-intelligence-in-wildlife-conservation-5dc3af2b4222.

tions vieillissant et fragile.[17] L'IA n'est pas parfaite sous tous rapports et de considérables développements sont nécessaires afin d'éviter un échec aussi retentissant que celui du robot Tay, mais des emplois courants de l'AI ont également rencontré un réel succès. Dans le milieu médical certaines applications novatrices de l'IA ne dérogent pas à la règle. En effet, des tentatives furent plus concluantes que d'autres, mais en somme l'IA au sens large a continué de s'imposer dans le domaine de la santé. C'est d'ailleurs à travers cette tendance dans le milieu médical que l'emploi de l'IA, même s'il s'était avéré concluant, a commencé à soulever des problèmes éthiques. Ces inquiétudes ne cessent d'augmenter alors que l'IA a se rapproche peu à peu du côté fort et que les systèmes d'IA ont commencé à s'imposer dans des espaces précédemment consacrés au personnel clinicien humain. Dans cette superposition de pouvoirs il est inquiétant de considérer que l'IA pourrait remplacer un praticien, ce qui viendrait bousculer une éthique installée dans un cadre bien établi de principisme, soit la déontologie privilégiée dans la médecine moderne en particulier aux États-Unis.

Le travail de Beauchamp et Childress au sujet du principisme précise les contours d'un cadre éthique fondé sur la manière dont le clinicien interagit avec son patient. Les quatre principes de non-malfaisance, bienfaisance, justice et autonomie guident les interactions du clinicien avec le patient, ainsi que le soutien qu'il lui apporte et les soins qu'il lui prodigue.[18] Ainsi, la relation médecin-patient est à la source d'une pratique éthique de la médecine. À mesure que cette relation s'établit, elle s'accompagne d'un sentiment de confiance.[19] Comme il est dûment noté dans l'ouvrage intitulé The Principles of Biomedical Ethics, « rien n'est plus important dans le système hospitalier que le maintien d'une culture de la confiance. »[20] La littérature scientifique évoquée plus loin dans ce travail indique aussi que les inquiétudes liées à l'introduction de l'IA dans le milieu médical sont fondées sur des problèmes de confiance, telle la crainte qu'un patient ne puisse pas prêter foi à des diagnostics, à des traitements ou à des interactions émanant d'une entité de l'IA. Ces inquiétudes se sont manifestées à

---

17. Gary Polakovic, "The next Big Effort in AI: Keeping L.A.'s Water Flowing Post-Earthquake," *USC News*, October 4, 2019, https://news.usc.edu/160680/ai-la-water-supply-earthquake-usc-research/.

18. Thomas L. Beauchamp and James F. Childress, *Principles of Biomedical Ethics*. New York: Oxford University Press, 2013.

19. Mark A. Hall et al., "Trust in Physicians and Medical Institutions: What Is It, Can It Be Measured, and Does It Matter?," *The Milbank Quarterly* 79, no. 4 (2001): 613.

20. Beauchamp and Childress, *Principles*, 40

travers les emplois historiques de l'IA en médecine, et ce dès les premières recherches effectuées dans ce domaine.

Dans les années 1970 le domaine de la santé a pu entrevoir ses premières mises en application des outils technologiques de l'IA. MYCIN, un des tout premiers systèmes d'IA mis au point par les chercheurs de l'école de médecine de Stanford, était employé pour identifier certaines bactéries, dont celles de la méningite et de la bactériémie, ainsi que pour proposer des traitements visant à la prévention des infections graves.[21] Plus d'une décennie avant l'invention d'internet, MYCIN était en mesure de proposer un protocole de soin obtenant un seuil d'acceptabilité de 65% selon les paramètres de cette étude. Par souci de comparaison, il fut demandé à cinq membres de la faculté d'élaborer un protocole de soin fondé sur les mêmes données, ce qui fit chuter les taux d'acceptabilité dans une fourchette comprise entre 42,5% et 62,5%. Même avec des résultats si prometteurs, l'éthique de l'emploi du système MYCIN fut immédiatement remis en cause dû au fait que le traitement individualisé était déterminé par affectation de probabilités plutôt que par un praticien.[22] En résumé, comment une machine pouvait-elle créer un protocole adapté à un cas clinique sans avoir aucune relation avec le patient et donc, aucune possibilité de déterminer quel traitement serait efficace ? En dépit du fait que MYCIN ne fut jamais mis en service dans le domaine de la santé, ces questions fondamentales persistèrent alors que l'IA continuait ses avancées en s'implantant peu à peu dans le cadre médical.

Les tentatives les plus prévalentes visant à entremêler IA et médecine occidentale moderne sont représentées dans les systèmes d'aide à la décision clinique (SADC), en particulier les systèmes d'aide au diagnostic médical (SADM). L'intention première dissimulée derrière l'emploi des SADM est d'interpréter des données afin de venir en aide au clinicien. L'assistance par recours au SADM pourrait, en théorie, aider un praticien à diagnostiquer un problème de santé en identifiant les manifestations et les signes avant-coureurs d'affections données afin de les signaler à un clinicien.[23] À présent,

---

21. V. L. Yu, "Antimicrobial Selection by a Computer. A Blinded Evaluation by Infectious Diseases Experts," *JAMA: The Journal of the American Medical Association* 242, no. 12 (1979): 1279–282.

22. David E. Heckerman, and Edward H. Shortliffe, "From Certainty Factors to Belief Networks," *Artificial Intelligence in Medicine* 4, no. 1 (1992): 37.

23. Eta S. Berner and Tonya J. La Lande, "Overview of Clinical Decision Support Systems," in *Clinical Decision Support Systems: Theory and Practice*, ed. Eta S. Berner (Switzerland: Springer International Press, 2016), 3.

la discipline la plus influencée par le SADM est la radiologie, étant donné l'application qui est faite de la technologie à l'imagerie médicale dont l'IRM et le tomodensitogramme. Les méthodes traditionnelles d'interprétation d'images médicales peuvent causer des erreurs de diagnostic, ce qui soulève la nécessité d'obtenir un second avis médical pouvant parfois venir compliquer le cas.[24] De plus, ces méthodes traditionnelles sont à la source d'une fatigue accrue des cliniciens tout en contribuant à une perte d'exactitude des diagnostics au cours de la journée de travail.[25] Les SADM qui ont déjà été développés et ceux qui se verront bientôt mis en service dans le cadre médical sont censés maîtriser certains de ces obstacles en donnant une seconde opinion en temps réel. Ainsi, le SADM peut prendre le relai du clinicien en proposant des suggestions dans de nombreux cas, sachant qu'il incombe au clinicien de prendre les décisions quant au diagnostic et au traitement préconisé.

Ayant décidé de tabler sur un certain engouement lié à l'inclusion totale du SADM dans le cadre médical, la société IBM a sorti un des exemples les plus célèbres d'IA au service du diagnostic médical : l'IA Watson dédiée au diagnostic des cancers. Le Watson d'IBM, ordinateur en mesure de comprendre le langage naturel et son contenu, connut un perfectionnement bien au-delà de ses ambitions premières afin de pouvoir prétendre à son utilisation dans le milieu médical.[26] Watson était conçu à l'origine pour se mesurer à des candidats humains au jeu télévisé du *Jeopardy !* Il remporta le succès en gagnant en 2011[27] contre Ken Jennings qui détenait le record du plus grand nombre de victoires consécutives au *Jeopardy !* de tous les temps. À la suite de cette victoire publique des outils technologiques de l'IA, IBM orienta les nouveaux objectifs de Watson vers la médecine en commercialisant en 2016 l'IA Watson for Oncology, dédiée au diagnostic des cancers.[28] Censé constituer la nouvelle limite de la médecine, Watson

24. Christopher Eakins et al., "Second Opinion Interpretations by Specialty Radiologists at a Pediatric Hospital: Rate of Disagreement and Clinical Implications," *American Journal of Roentgenology* 199, no. 4 (2012): pp. 916-920.
25. Elizabeth A. Krupinski et al., "Long Radiology Workdays Reduce Detection and Accommodation Accuracy," *Journal of the American College of Radiology* 7, no. 9 (2010): pp. 698–704
26. IBM, "Watson Overview," The DeepQA Research Team, July 25, 2016, https://researcher.watson.ibm.com/researcher/view_group.php?id=2099.
27. Eric Brown, "Watson: The *Jeopardy*^! Challenge and beyond," 2013 *IEEE 12th International Conference on Cognitive Informatics and Cognitive Computing*, 2013.
28. IBM Newsroom, "Manipal Hospitals Announces National Launch of IBM Watson for Oncology," July 26, 2016, https://www-03.ibm.com/press/in/en/pressrelease/50290.wss.

était présenté comme un système d'IA en mesure non seulement d'assister à l'interprétation d'images médicales, mais également capable de proposer un traitement véritablement efficace sans l'aval d'un clinicien. Les défenseurs de l'IA y virent une manière de prouver que la mise en service d'outils d'IA plus avancés en médecine avait ses bénéfices. Néanmoins, des considérations éthiques concernant une machine en capacité de prendre des décisions furent sujet à controverse.[29] Comme on l'apprit plus tard en s'appuyant sur des documents internes à la société IBM rendus publics en juillet 2018, une grande partie de ces craintes concernant l'emploi de Watson était légitime.

Une enquête du quotidien The Boston Globe, STAT révéla que les cadres d'IBM étaient au fait des problèmes du système de diagnostic oncologique Watson, soulignant que celui-ci avait livré « en de multiples occurrences des recommandations inadéquates et risquées. »[30] La plupart de ces problèmes n'étaient pas non plus inconnus des employés d'IBM. En effet, des archives révèlent les tentatives d'IBM de contacter des cliniciens pour les avertir que Watson disposait de capacités « très limitées ».[31] Ces tentatives demeurèrent sans succès permettant aux systèmes installés dans les hôpitaux de continuer à fonctionner selon la présomption que Watson for Oncology était capable de proposer des possibilités de traitement aux patients. À l'issue du rapport du STAT dévoilant les protocoles de soin inadaptés émis par Watson, de nombreux hôpitaux publièrent rapidement des démentis ayant pour but de dissiper les craintes selon lesquelles l'IA était allée trop loin, remplaçant effectivement le clinicien dans sa prise de décision clinique. Dans une déclaration censée rassurer l'opinion publique, déclaration soutenant que Watson n'avait été employé que comme un outil de diagnostic et non comme une entité investie d'un pouvoir décisionnaire, le porte-parole d'un hôpital déclara : « Aucune invention technologique ne peut remplacer un médecin ou sa connaissance intime du cas de chaque patient. »[32] Le message était clair : la relation médecin-patient n'était en aucun cas ternie par l'utilisation de Watson for Oncology puisque les cliniciens ne faisaient pas usage de ce système d'aide au diagnostic pour prendre des décisions importantes.

---

29. Jennifer Bresnick, "Artificial Intelligence in Healthcare Market to See 40% CAGR Surge," HealthITAnalytics, July 24, 2017, https://healthitanalytics.com/news/artificial-intelligence-in-healthcare-market-to-see-40-cagr-surge.
30. Casey Ross and Ike Swetlitz, "IBM's Watson supercomputer recommended 'unsafe and incorrect' cancer treatments, internal documents show," *STAT*, July 25, 2018.
31. Julie Spitzer, "IBM's Watson recommended 'unsafe and incorrect' cancer treatments, STAT report finds," *Becker's Healthcare*, July 25, 2018.
32. Spitzer, "IBM's Watson."

En d'autres mots, ces décisions demeuraient entièrement à la discrétion du clinicien. Toutefois, même après que l'exactitude de diagnostic de Watson a été remise en question, le logiciel est encore employé dans les systèmes hospitaliers à ce jour, à compter les soixante-dix Centres médicaux des vétérans, les Veterans Affairs Medical Centers, aux États-Unis.[33]

L'usage ininterrompu de Watson for Oncology n'est pas le seul signe indiquant que les organismes de santé sont toujours intéressés par une découverte des fonctions possibles de l'IA en médecine. Il est vrai que le diagnostic assisté par IA a été mis en service avec la garantie que le clinicien serait toujours en pleine possession de ses décisions médicales, mais à ce moment-même des entreprises sont en train de développer des outils technologiques dotés d'IA, leur faisant ainsi une place de plus en plus prépondérante dans le domaine médical. À un tel point que des préoccupations très sérieuses se sont en réalité imposées au sujet de l'IA employée en remplacement de cliniciens.[34] Et le constat est clair : au jour d'aujourd'hui, de nombreux programmes informatiques ont même été capables de réussir leurs études de médecine.

En 2017, la Chine fut le tout premier pays à être témoin de la réussite d'une IA aux examens de médecine. Un robot intelligent nommé Xiaoyi, ce qui en mandarin veut dire "le petit docteur », a défrayé la chronique pour avoir obtenu le score de 456 points sur 600 aux examens de médecine chinois, soient 96 points de plus que la note minimale d'admission.[35] Il faut savoir qu'il est impossible de réussir à l'examen chinois par seul recours à la mémorisation. En effet, cet examen est structuré de telle manière que les médecins en devenir doivent se livrer à des études de cas et donc, décider quelle réponse y apporter selon les informations à disposition. Cette épreuve est censée prouver que les candidats sont capables d'interpréter les données médicales qui leur sont présentées afin de prendre une décision sensée et éclairée.[36] La première tentative de Xiaoyi s'étant soldée par un échec (avec

33. Eliza Strickland, "How IBM Watson Overpromised and Underdelivered on AI Health Care," *IEEE Spectrum: Technology, Engineering, and Science News*, April 2, 2019, https://spectrum.ieee.org/biomedical/diagnostics/how-ibm-watson-overpromised-and-underdelivered-on-ai-health-care.

34. Kyle E. Karches, "Against the iDoctor: Why Artificial Intelligence Should Not Replace Physician Judgment," *Theoretical Medicine and Bioethics* 39 (2): 92

35. Ma Si, and Cheng Yu, "Chinese Robot Becomes World's First Machine to Pass Medical Exam," *China Daily*, November 10, 2017, http://www.chinadaily.com.cn/business/tech/2017-11/10/content_34362656.htm.

36. Alice Yan, "How a Robot Passed China's Medical Licensing Exam," *South China Morning Post*, November 20, 2017, accessed April 20, 2019.

un score à peine au-dessus de 100) donne une idée du réel niveau de difficulté de l'examen. Avant sa deuxième tentative, l'équipe de chercheurs
avait forcé Xiaoyi à « étudier » en présentant au robot de nombreux ouvrages
médicaux ainsi que des cas d'école.[37] Comme les autres candidats ayant
réussi l'examen à cette période, Xiaoyi devait se préparer à l'épreuve écrite.
Cependant, quand Xiaoyi montra qu'il était bien renseigné sur de nombreux
types d'affections, l'équipe de chercheurs fut prompte à annoncer qu'il était
seulement capable de « faire des suggestions aux médecins afin de les aider
à identifier des problèmes au plus vite et d'ainsi éviter certains risques. »[38]
En dépit du fait que cette IA avait réussi à l'examen de médecine, il valait
mieux être clair avec les patients en leur garantissant qu'ils recevraient des
soins aux mains de médecins et non d'une IA.

Une tout autre réaction a pu être constatée la fois suivante où une IA a
réussi à l'examen de médecine. C'est en juin 2018 que l'IA Babylon Health
a réussi l'examen britannique du Royal College of General Practitioners
(MRCGP). Le MRCGP est le dernier d'une série d'examens censés évaluer
les connaissances des candidats dans la spécialisation qu'ils comptent briguer.
En somme, la réussite au MRCGP indique qu'à l'issue de nombreuses
années d'étude le candidat est fin prêt à pratiquer la médecine. Le score
moyen obtenu à cet examen de 2012 à 2017 était de 72%, à savoir que l'IA
Babylon a été reçu avec un score de 81%.[39] Dans un communiqué publié
après le succès de l'IA de la société Babylon, son fondateur et PDG, le Dr.
Ali Parsa, contrairement à ses confrères, ne prit pas la peine de se vouloir
rassurant quant au fait que le but de cette technologie n'était pas de remplacer
les cliniciens ni de prendre des décisions médicales directement avec un
patient. Soulignant le fait que la possibilité de voir un clinicien est parfois
très limitée et les systèmes de santé surchargés, le Dr. Parsa affirma que cet
accomplissement de l'IA à travers sa réussite à l'examen du MRCGP était
« une illustration claire de la manière dont les services de santé fonctionnant
avec l'IA pourraient soulager les charges pesant sur les systèmes de santé
dans le monde entier. »[40] Ce succès de l'IA Babylon marque un basculement
de la rhétorique au sujet de l'emploi de l'IA en médecine : son futur rôle
pourrait ne pas se limiter à celui d'un outil consultable par les cliniciens,
mais bien suppléer le clinicien lui-même.

---

37. Si and Yu, "Chinese Robot."
38. Yan, "How a Robot."
39. Babylon Health, "Babylon AI Achieves Equivalent Accuracy with Human Doctors in Global Healthcare First," *PR Newswire: News Distribution, Targeting and Monitoring,* June 27, 2018.
40. Babylon Health, "Babylon AI Achieves Equivalent Accuracy with Human Doctors."

Des changements récents dans le domaine médical ont montré que les perspectives d'avenir évoquées par le Dr. Parsa pourraient bien prendre corps. Actuellement, un secteur de la médecine progresse de manière exponentielle, la télémédecine, dont le développement s'accompagne de conversations quant à l'évolution de la pratique médicale envers les patients.[41] Aux États-Unis, la téléconsultation, définie dans une étude de l'American Hospital Association en tant que « vidéoconférence, surveillance à distance, consultations électroniques, et communications sans fil », qui est proposée aux patients par l'intermédiaire de leur système de santé a augmenté de 35% à 76% de 2010 à 2017.[42] Un aspect commun de la télémédecine est la possibilité de prendre des rendez-vous médicaux virtuels, tels que ceux proposés par la clinique de Cleveland, dont le but est de traiter des affections bénignes ne nécessitant pas de rendez-vous en personne telles le rhume, les allergies et même la grippe, ce qui est précisément le type de consultation auquel faisait référence le Dr. Parsa dans son communiqué au sujet des applications possibles de l'IA Babylon.[43]

Les patients américains commencent à s'habituer à l'idée de prendre un conseil médical ainsi que de se voir prescrire un traitement par le biais de la technologie. Des exemples dans notre pays et dans le monde démontrent que les individus sont disposés à interagir avec un humain par l'intermédiaire d'un outil technologique, et même voir les technologies de l'IA remplacer des cliniciens. Un des exemples les plus importants dans la pratique médicale actuelle est l'emploi des robots conversationnels thérapeutiques. Il a été mis en évidence que ces agents conversationnels aident les patients à mieux comprendre le diagnostic qui leur est fait ainsi qu'à adhérer au protocole de soin correspondant.[44] Une autre étude montre que les patient atteints d'un stress post-traumatique étaient plus ouverts à la communication et capables de reconnaître leur traumatisme en décrivant leurs symptômes à un robot plutôt qu'à une personne.[45] Cependant, on n'en est pas au point où cette version de l'IA dans le domaine médical s'apprêterait déjà à remplacer les modèles thérapeutiques en place.

---

41. Tommaso Iannitti et al., "Narrative Review of Telemedicine Consultation in Medical Practice," *Patient Preference and Adherence*, 2015, 65.
42. American Hospital Association, "Fact Sheet: Telehealth," February 2019.
43. "Cleveland Clinic Express Care® Online," Cleveland Clinic, 2019.
44. Aditya Vaidyam and John Torous. "Chatbots: What Are They and Why Care?" *Psychiatric Times*, June 27, 2019. https://www.psychiatrictimes.com/telepsychiatry/chatbots-what-are-they-and-why-care.
45. Myrthe L. Tielman et al., "A Therapy System for Post-Traumatic Stress Disorder Using a Virtual Agent and Virtual Storytelling to Reconstruct Traumatic Memories," *Journal of Medical Systems* 41, no. 8 (2017): 125.

Alors que les participants à ces études ont bien voulu parler à un robot à qui ils ont d'ailleurs révélé plus de détails qu'ils ne le feraient en personne au premier abord ou lors d'une visioconférence, la recherche démontre qu'il existe à cela quelques réserves. En particulier, des études indiquent que certains individus sont désireux de communiquer plus d'informations à un de ces agents conversationnels intelligents quand ils sont assurés qu'un clinicien lira la transcription des échanges.[46] Cela étant dit, même si les participants étaient rassurés de savoir qu'ils obtiendraient un diagnostic psychologique solide ou un retour thérapeutique d'un clinicien en chair et en os, ils étaient tout de même désireux de se confier à une IA au début de la démarche thérapeutique pendant la session initiale. Considérant le succès commercial des applications de santé mentale et le fait que l'Association Américaine de Psychiatrie a commencé à catégoriser et à évaluer l'efficacité potentielle de ces applications, lesquelles contiennent souvent une composante conversationnelle, il est tout à fait raisonnable de penser que le public en fera plus d'usage à l'avenir.[47]

L'idée même du thérapeute virtuel impose une dynamique différente de celle du modèle traditionnel, même si un clinicien est appelé à intervenir à la fin du processus. Dans ce nouveau modèle, la relation médecin-patient prend un aspect différent des interactions face-à-face, d'humain à humain décrites par Beauchamp et Childress. Bien que les participants aient voulu s'assurer que la prise de décision médicale restait aux mains d'un humain, la construction de la relation était initialement laissée à une IA. Cela marque une divergence d'approche par rapport à celles qu'on avait pu constater dans le cas des systèmes d'aide au diagnostic médical (SADM) comme Watson for Oncology qui opère en coulisses. Ces systèmes d'IA sont d'ailleurs conçus pour être employés comme des outils intervenant en toute discrétion pour établir un diagnostic en corrélation avec l'expertise d'un clinicien. Un agent conversationnel virtuel conçu à des fins thérapeutiques interagit en premier avec l'humain et relaie ensuite les renseignements rassemblés lors de l'échange d'un prestataire humain à un autre. L'IA de ces robots conversationnels thérapeutiques ne prend pas d'images, mais fait un travail fondé sur le dialogue et la relation avec un client. Cette relation pourrait

---

46. Timothy W. Bickmore et al., "Response to a Relational Agent by Hospital Patients with Depressive Symptoms," *Interacting with Computers* 22, no. 4 (2010): 289.
47. Jessica Truschel, "Top 25 Mental Health Apps for 2020: An Alternative to Therapy?," Psycom.net– Mental Health Treatment Resource Since 1986, March 19, 2020, https://www.psycom.net/25-best-mental-health-apps.

ne pas porter de ressemblance avec celle qui anime le tandem clinicien-patient mis en place par la médecine moderne, mais dans ces circonstances précises, l'IA est indéniablement mêlée à la relation entre le patient et le médecin. Et alors que ces agents conversationnels intelligents ne peuvent visiblement pas remplacer une interaction en personne avec un clinicien, d'autres outils technologiques en cours d'élaboration dans les laboratoires scientifiques du monde entier cherchent à repousser cette limite.

Au Japon où l'IA fait l'objet d'une perception très positive, les technologies de l'IA qui accompagnent les patients de manière directe vont plus loin que les thérapies en ligne. En effet, le Japon a commencé à mettre en service des robots de soin équipés d'IA qui sont capables de dispenser un dosage approprié de médicaments et de subvenir aux besoins de base de leur population de seniors, par exemple en réglant la température dans leur chambre.[48] La demande d'outils robotiques a tant augmenté dans les soins gériatriques que de nombreuses entreprises automobiles ont converti leurs activités, passant ainsi de la conception de véhicules autonomes aux géronto-technologies, telles les lits transformables en chaises roulantes ou l'emploi de supports cybernétiques, permettant au personnel de soin de soulever les patients sans aide extérieure.[49] De manière plus directe et plus personnelle, les robots humanoïdes équipés d'IA, tel Pepper construit par SoftBank Robotics, ont été conçus pour chanter des chansons aux patients âgés et pour répondre à des questions simples comme « où se trouvent les toilettes ? »[50] Même les animaux de compagnie conçus au Japon, tel le phoque robotisé Paro, ont été inventés spécifiquement pour réagir aux interactions humaines donnant ainsi les moyens aux patients âgés de construire une relation avec une entité non-vivante.[51]

Les outils technologiques comme Paro et Pepper ont obtenu un grand succès, car ils ont été conçus à dessein pour capitaliser sur l'habilité culturelle unique des patients japonais à créer des liens avec une IA. Étant donné l'à priori favorable qu'ont les Japonais envers l'IA, il n'est pas étonnant que leur culture soit très en avance quant à son adoption en médecine. Dans les exemples cités, les outils technologiques étaient mis en service pour

---

48. Naomi Tajitsu, "Japanese Automakers Look to Robots to Aid the Elderly," *Scientific American*. April 12, 2017, https://www.scientificamerican.com/article/japanese-automakers-look-to-robots-to-aid-the-elderly.
49. Don Lee, "Desperate for Workers."
50. Don Lee, "Desperate for Workers."
51. Amy Harmon, "A Soft Spot for Circuitry," *The New York Times*. July 5, 2010, https://www.nytimes.com/2010/07/05/science/05robot.html?_r=2&pagewanted=1.

assurer les soins des seniors tout en palliant le manque de personnel médical. En utilisant les outils mis à disposition par l'IA en médecine, les robots humanoïdes japonais dotés d'IA satisfont à cette première condition énoncée, et ce, de manière éthique. La seconde condition qui consiste à assurer le maintien de la relation patient-clinicien s'en voit partiellement satisfaite, vu que les patients ont fait montre d'une habilité claire à créer un lien avec ces outils, quoique différemment de la manière classique impliquant le patient et le clinicien qui prend les décisions médicales. Bien que l'IA humanoïde japonaise n'atteigne pas complètement le niveau des technologies futures qui pourraient être mises en service dans le domaine de la santé à l'avenir, les outils actuels constituent certainement un pas dans cette direction.

En substance, les États-Unis ne sont probablement pas prêts à une mise en service à grande échelle d'humanoïdes équipés d'IA semblables à ceux que l'on voit au Japon. Tout au plus, les technologies de l'IA les plus facilement adaptables au système de santé américain ressembleraient probablement à l'IA de Babylon où l'intelligence artificielle agirait en tant que clinicien en première ligne de soin. En tant que telle, l'IA serait en mesure d'établir un diagnostic rapide sur des affections bénignes comme les rhumes et les grippes, envoyant le patient à un clinicien en cas de besoin. Une IA de ce calibre pourrait tout à fait être mise en service aux États-Unis en adhérant aux deux principes éthiques suivants, à savoir satisfaire aux exigences d'un cas documenté et maintenir la relation patient-clinicien.

Le système de santé américain connaît les mêmes besoins que ceux qui sont pris en charge par l'IA au Japon, tout au moins concernant les préoccupations liées à une population vieillissante. Toutefois, l'inquiétude monte aux États-Unis concernant un manque de soutien accessible aux patients âgés ; cette inquiétude a été relayée dans un rapport datant de mars 2019 publié par le gouvernement Trump.[52] Le rapport intitulé Emerging Technologies to Support an Aging Population (Technologies émergentes destinées au soin des aînés) indique clairement que le modèle de santé actuel ne fonctionne pas et que des technologies émergentes devraient être prises en compte afin de soulager le fardeau incombant aux prestataires de soins de santé. En adoptant certains outils technologiques, les États-Unis deviendraient moins dépendants des aides aux soins de santé à domicile, type d'emploi en forte croissance dû au nombre de gens nécessitant ce type de soins. Or, des

---

52. Mark Mather, Paola Scommegna, and Lillian Kilduff, "Fact Sheet: Aging in the United States," Population Reference Bureau, July 15, 2019, https://www.prb.org/aging-unitedstates-fact-sheet/.

inquiétudes liées à la faible rémunération et aux demandes physiques de ce type d'emploi sont en passe de contribuer à une pénurie dans cette catégorie de personnel à domicile.[53] A savoir que le manque de personnel ne touche certainement pas que les États-Unis où l'on remarque des insuffisances de soins qui pourraient être allégées ou résolues grâce à la technologie.

Les populations rurales constituent un défi particulier pour le système de santé dans son modèle moderne. Avec ses centres hospitaliers centralisés établis dans les plus grandes villes de la nation, les cliniciens se sont éloignés de l'image idéale du médecin de campagne pouvant effectuer des visites à domicile. Les défis apportés par les patients vivant dans des régions reculées a fait augmenter le besoin de solutions impliquant la télémédecine.[54] Lorsqu'il est donné aux patients la possibilité de voir un médecin virtuellement, ceux-ci n'ont pas à faire le trajet pour rejoindre l'établissement de soins le plus proche, ni à trouver un moyen de transport quand ils n'ont pas de véhicule personnel à disposition ou ne peuvent compter sur la visite d'un médecin. La société Babylon Health, par exemple, cible ouvertement les patients vivant dans ces zones isolées. Après sa réussite à l'examen de médecine au Royaume-Uni, l'IA de la société Babylon fut d'abord distribuée à des populations isolées d'Afrique permettant à un système de santé marqué par un manque de cliniciens de proposer des consultations à un plus grand nombre de patients et surtout de passer plus de temps auprès de ceux nécessitant des soins particuliers.[55] La société Babylon basée à Londres s'est beaucoup développée depuis grâce au système d'exploitation iOS et à une application Android censée offrir la même médecine de première ligne à tous les gens possédant un smartphone aux États-Unis. L'idée maîtresse de cette technologie est simple : dans un système où l'accès à la santé constitue un défi, il s'agit de trouver un moyen de faciliter cet accès.

Si l'IA en tant que clinicien de première ligne peut interagir avec un patient et diagnostiquer des maladies communes et des affections comme les allergies, le rhume, ou même la grippe, alors l'interaction médecin-patient peut en théorie être réservée aux cas plus complexes. Etant donné que le clinicien n'aurait pas besoin d'accorder du temps aux patients dont

53. U.S. Bureau of Labor Statistics, "Home Health Aides and Personal Care Aides: Occupational Outlook Handbook," September 4, 2019. https://www.bls.gov/ooh/healthcare/home-health-aides-and-personal-care-aides.htm.
54. Ahmed Hosny and Hugo J. W. L. Aerts, "Artificial Intelligence for Global Health." American Association for the Advancement of Science, November 22, 2019, https://science.sciencemag.org/content/366/6468/955.full.
55. Babylon Health, "Babylon AI Achieves Equivalent Accuracy with Human Doctors."

les affections peuvent être diagnostiquées de façon rapide et facile grâce à l'IA, il serait alors disponible pour avoir une conversation plus longue et plus détaillée avec des patients ayant besoin de soins plus spécifiques. Non seulement cela permettrait de maintenir une relation patient-clinicien entre un humain et une IA de première ligne pouvant prendre des décisions médicales, mais cela pourrait aussi optimiser la relation humaine médecin-patient. Toutefois, le modèle dans lequel l'IA prend la décision médicale a été vivement critiqué, même pour des diagnostics simples : il s'agit d'un phénomène connu sous le nom de boîte noire. L'inquiétude qu'il soulève est la suivante : dans l'éventualité où le diagnostic proviendrait d'une IA, même si la décision médicale semblait logique, il est impossible pour un humain de comprendre de quelle manière le diagnostic a été rendu.[56]

Le fait que l'IA fonctionne sur le principe de la boîte noire peut être source de frustration étant donné l'impossibilité intrinsèque de comprendre ce qui fait une décision prise par IA, et par le fait que ce sentiment est probablement né de pratiques médicales anciennes liées aux relations médecin-patient. D'ailleurs, l'effet boîte noire pose un problème éthique semblable à celui que l'on peut constater dans certaines approches paternalistes de la médecine en ce que l'IA prend une décision que le patient est supposé accepter sans discuter. Avec les progrès de la médecine, on a pu constater parmi les patients dans les systèmes de santé occidentaux un désir accru d'autonomie dans la décision médicale et d'un certain contrôle sur les soins qu'ils veulent se voir prodiguer.[57] Cependant, il est possible que les technologies futures soient libérées de ces contraintes avec les progrès de l'IA. Cette dernière peut bien rendre une décision, mais si le problème de la boîte noire est pris en considération au plus vite, il est fort possible que des chercheurs concevront les technologies de la future IA afin qu'elles soient en capacité d'expliquer pourquoi certaines conclusions ont été retenues selon des données précises. Un tel progrès constituerait une remarquable impulsion partant d'une IA faible pour aller vers une IA forte, et au vu des exemples concernant les systèmes de diagnostic et les systèmes d'IA capables de réussir médecine, il est évident que des pas vers cette tendance sont déjà en train de se concrétiser.

Sans vouloir tomber dans le débat concernant un paternalisme potentiel au sein de l'IA et des habitudes paternalistes ancrées chez les cliniciens qui

---

56. Robin C. Feldman, Ehrik Aldana, and Kara Stein. 2019. "Artificial Intelligence in the Health Care Space: How can we trust what we cannot know," *Stanford Law & Policy Review* 30 (2): 406.
57. Beauchamp and Childress, *Principles*, 220.

visent la bienfaisance, il y a un point supplémentaire à ajouter suggérant que la boîte noire ne doit pas être considérée comme un défaut majeur des technologies de l'IA. Pour le dire simplement, le fait qu'une IA ne soit pas capable d'expliquer à un patient les tenants et les aboutissants d'une prise de décision concernant sa santé peut être mis en parallèle avec le cas d'un spécialiste tentant d'expliquer les tenants et les aboutissants d'un raisonnement médical à un patient n'ayant aucune connaissance de la médecine. Par ailleurs, les manques de communication et les incompréhensions entre cliniciens et patients sont bien documentés dans la littérature médicale, ce qui indique que même si un médecin a théoriquement les moyens d'expliquer ses décisions, il ne le fait pas toujours avec précision ou rigueur.[58] Tout cela révèle, cependant, que peu importe si c'est un clinicien ou une IA qui pose le diagnostic directement au patient, car il faut avant tout éviter les erreurs de communication et maintenir la confiance entre le patient et son médecin. Avec le développement des systèmes d'IA, des chercheurs devraient faire en sorte d'atténuer le problème de la boîte noire, quoique son existence au sein de l'IA n'indique pas en soi que cette technologie soit indubitablement caractérisée par un manque d'éthique.

Il est à parier que, dans un avenir où le problème de la boîte noire sera résolu, où la société sera à même d'accorder sa pleine confiance à une décision prise par IA sans demander d'explication, des problèmes liés à l'utilisation de l'IA perdureront. Une des inquiétudes premières des individus ayant choisi de se reposer sur l'IA plutôt que sur leur propre savoir-faire réside dans le fait qu'ils pourraient être tentés de mettre de côté leur propre intelligence pour dépendre à tort de la technologie. Un exemple de ce phénomène est celui de conducteurs qui, en suivant aveuglément les instructions de leur GPS, précipitèrent leur véhicule dans une étendue d'eau.[59] À chaque fois, ces personnes ont visiblement préféré mettre de côté leur propre sens de l'orientation, ignorant les panneaux de direction qui indiquaient qu'ils n'étaient pas sur le bon chemin et décidant de suivre les instructions de leur GPS envers et contre tout jusqu'à la submersion. En général, ces situations n'ont pas fait de blessés et n'ont occasionné que des dommages matériels, un sentiment d'humiliation et quelques gros titres dans les journaux. Pourtant,

---

58. Dennis Rosen. *Vital Conversations: Improving Communication Between Doctors and Patients.* New York: Columbia University Press, 2014, 161–162.
59. Malone Kircher. "Yet Another Person Listens to GPS App and Drives Car into Lake." *Intelligencer*, January 24, 2018. https://nymag.com/intelligencer/2018/01/waze-app-directs-driver-to-drive-car-into-lake-champlain.html.

dans certains cas, la dépendance à un outil technologique défectueux peut avoir des conséquences bien moins bénignes. Dans le cas de Watson for Oncology, il a vite été clair que les traitements envisagés ne seraient pas efficaces pour certains patients, et pouvaient ainsi faire plus de mal que de bien. Des patients auraient pu perdre la vie si les cliniciens s'en étaient remis uniquement aux suggestions de l'IA au lieu de compter sur leur formation médicale afin de repérer des cas où un traitement n'était pas approprié. À savoir que les informations erronées provenant d'une IA et de la confiance aveugle d'un clinicien en une IA qui « savait mieux » que lui auraient été la cause directe de ces décès.

Le problème de la boîte noire et l'éventualité qu'un clinicien puisse laisser de côté sa formation médicale pour s'en référer uniquement à une IA adoptée par un système de santé sont certainement des problèmes à prendre en compte puisque l'IA est de plus en plus mêlée à la prise de décision médicale. Néanmoins, ces préoccupations ne devraient pas empêcher le recours aux technologies futures au sein des systèmes de santé. En acceptant cet état de fait au vu des tendances actuelles qui marquent les technologies de l'IA dans le monde et aux États-Unis, il est impératif d'envisager les applications éthiques des technologies qui pourront s'inscrire dans un avenir proche. Comme il a été évoqué plus haut, la prochaine étape logique de l'emploi de l'IA dans le domaine de la santé est celle du rôle qu'elle pourrait assumer en tant que clinicien de première ligne. En cela, il faut garder en mémoire que le recours éthique aux systèmes d'IA en médecine est à double ressort : l'IA doit combler un besoin dans l'environnement médical et le patient doit être capable d'établir un lien avec l'IA de façon à ce que la relation médecin-patient soit préservée. Certains cabinets médicaux ou quelque secteur d'un système hospitalier donné pourraient assumer quelques aspects de ces critères, mais il existe un système de santé aux États-Unis qui serait visiblement susceptible de constituer, dans sa totalité, le fondement d'une utilisation éthique de l'IA en première ligne de soin : il s'agit de l'administration des anciens combattants, la Veterans Health Administration (VHA).

Afin d'établir la nécessité du recours éthique à l'IA pour le diagnostic médical dans ce contexte particulier, il faut savoir que la VHA s'est rendue tristement célèbre par de longs délais d'attente, des soins inadéquats et la réputation de ne pas répondre aux besoins de ses patients. Les démarches nécessaires à l'obtention de la couverture de santé proposée par la VHA peuvent tourner au cauchemar pour certains membres des forces armées américaines auxquels ces services sont pourtant réservés. Parmi des exemples particulièrement atroces liés à une mauvaise gestion des demandes de prestations d'invalidité, il y a celui d'un garde côte blessé pendant son service qui a passé trente-quatre ans à faire appel de son droit à l'allocation handicapé auprès du département des anciens combattants.[60] Dans un cas similaire, une ancienne combattante souffrant de diabète a dû lutter pour ses droits aux soins, encourant pendant ce temps l'amputation d'un pied ; avant que sa demande ait été approuvée, la double amputation était consommée.[61] À savoir que même lorsqu'un vétéran se voit octroyer ses droits, des problèmes sérieux subsistent.

La VHA est tristement renommée pour les difficultés que connaissent les anciens combattants dans la prise de rendez-vous médicaux dans un délai convenable, même pour les affections engageant leur pronostic vital.[62] Ce problème a fait la une des médias dans tous les États-Unis lorsque CNN a sorti un rapport au sujet du système de santé des anciens combattants de la ville de Phoenix, dans l'état de l'Arizona, où des vétérans ont perdu la vie pour n'avoir pas pu obtenir de consultation avec un médecin. CNN a mis en évidence que ces décès étaient le résultat d'une liste secrète créée par des administrateurs de la VHA pour dissimuler le fait qu'environ 1500 patients avaient été contraints d'attendre des mois avant d'obtenir un rendez-vous en consultation, ce qui a entraîné la mort d'environ quarante d'entre eux par défaut de soin.[63] La VHA a alors pris des mesures pour identifier des secteurs où l'attente dépasse la norme en vigueur concernant l'accès aux soins en temps utile, mais il est difficile de déterminer ce qui constitue une longue attente et de composer avec un système qui permet la prise de rendez-vous, mais finit par les reporter de nombreuses fois.[64] Il y a eu des progrès de faits depuis le scandale de Phoenix, mais l'attente reste un souci majeur pour la VHA, en dépit des mesures mises en place ces dernières

---

60. Dave Philipps, "Veterans Claiming Disability Pay Face Wall of Denials and Delays," *The New York Times*, November 13, 2017, https://www.nytimes.com/2017/11/13/us/veterans-affairs-department-benefits-delays.html.
61. Dave Phillips, "Veterans Claiming Disability Pay."
62. *Waiting for Care: Examining Patient Wait Times at VA Committee on Veterans' Affairs Committee on Veterans' Affairs*, 2013, Statement of Chairman Mike Coffman, Subcommittee on Oversight and Investigations of Veterans' Affairs. http://search.ebscohost.com/login.aspx?direct=true&AuthType=ip,shib&db=cat07006a&AN=cwru.b4081068&site=eds-live.
63. Scott Bronstein and Drew Griffin, "A Fatal Wait: Veterans Languish and Die on a VA Hospital's Secret List," *CNN* (Cable News Network, April 24, 2014), https://www.cnn.com/2014/04/23/health/veterans-dying-health-care-delays/index.html.
64. Brendan McGarry, "VA Audit Confirms Veterans' Wait Times Complaints," Military.com, 2014, https://www.military.com/daily-news/2014/06/10/va-audit-confirms-veterans-wait-times-complaints.html.

années pour améliorer les systèmes de prise de rendez-vous et accroître la surveillance des temps d'attente.[65] Alors que la prise de rendez-vous et son report fréquent sont cités comme une des raisons d'une longue attente, il faut aussi compter sur la pénurie de personnel de santé.

Des estimations suggèrent que d'ici 2025, une pénurie de cliniciens aux États-Unis affectera principalement les systèmes hospitaliers situés en milieu rural et ceux qui seront dans l'incapacité de proposer des salaires compétitifs.[66] Malheureusement, la VHA pêche par ces deux aspects, ce qui cause des inquiétudes supplémentaires pour les centres médicaux de l'administration des anciens combattants dont les subventions sont insuffisantes. Par ailleurs, de potentiels problèmes causés par une future pénurie de médecins ont déjà été repérés au sein de la VHA. Entre 2011 et 2015, le nombre de cliniciens quittant ce système de santé a augmenté chaque année à cause de départs en retraite et de démissions spontanées.[67] En 2018 l'office gouvernemental des comptes, la United States Government Accountability Office (GAO), a issu un rapport démontrant clairement que la VHA traverse des difficultés de recrutement et de rétention des médecins et bien que des mesures aient été prises pour améliorer la rétention, bon nombre de ses centres médicaux ne peuvent compter que sur des intervenants à mi-temps, sur des bénévoles ou sur les cliniciens en stage qui finissent par quitter également ce système de soins.[68] Naturellement, la VHA a fait du recrutement une de ses priorités, mais l'office gouvernemental des comptes a découvert en 2019 que les tentatives d'augmenter le nombre de médecins n'avaient réussi qu'au prix d'un défaut d'accréditation des cliniciens.[69] Dans un exemple flagrant cité dans le rapport en question, la VHA avait embauché un médecin dont la licence avait précédemment été révoquée pour préjudice porté à un patient par négligence. Par ailleurs, tous les rapports au sujet du temps d'attente, de la disponibilité et du recrutement des médecins brossent également le portrait d'une VHA en cruel manque de moyens.

---

65. Patricia Kime, "5 Years After Nationwide Scandal, VA Still Struggles to Track Wait Times," Military.com, July 26, 2019, https://www.military.com/daily-news/2019/07/26/5-years-after-nationwide-scandal-va-still-struggles-track-wait-times.html.
66. Department of Health and Human Services, Health Resources and Services Administration, Designated Health Professional Shortage Areas Statistic, HRSA Data Warehouse, 2017.
67. *Steps Taken to Improve Physician Staffing, Recruitment, and Retention, but Challenges Remain.* Statement by Director of Health Care, Debra Draper Before the Subcommittee on Health, Committee on Veterans' Affairs, House of Representatives Veterans Health, 2018.
68. *Steps Taken to Improve Physician Staffing.*
69. Kathy Larin, "Veterans health administration: Greater focus on credentialing needed to prevent disqualified providers from delivering patient care," *Nova Science Publishers, Inc.* 2019: 205.

Alors qu'une petite partie des défis auxquels fait face la VHA peuvent être résolus par le recours à l'IA, sa mise en service en tant que clinicien de première ligne soulagerait de nombreuses inquiétudes tout en assurant la première des deux conditions nécessaires à sa mise en place éthique. L'évocation d'une utilisation de l'IA dans ce contexte ne serait pas une première puisque que son emploi a déjà été présenté comme une solution aux problèmes logistiques de la VHA. En effet, en 2008, au cours d'une audience devant le comité des anciens combattants, le Committee on Veterans' Affairs, était présentée une proposition de recours à l'IA pour renforcer le système de traitement des demandes de soins de santé de la VHA.[70] En dépit du scandale de la VHA de Phoenix concernant le traitement des demandes de prestations, les propositions faites lors de cette audition ne produisirent pas les résultats escomptés. Toutefois, dès 2021, sera prévue la mise en service d'un nouveau système de logiciel, laquelle affectera toutes les antennes de la VHA, dans le but de sensiblement améliorer le processus de prise de rendez-vous de consultation et d'écourter l'attente.[71] Bien évidemment, il faudra du temps pour constater si l'adoption de l'IA dans le logiciel de prise de rendez-vous entraînera la diminution des plaintes déposées par des patients connaissant des difficultés à obtenir une consultation en temps utile. Quoique le système facilite le suivi, de la prise des rendez-vous à la confirmation, le problème de la pénurie de médecins qualifiés demeure et doit être pris en compte. L'emploi actuel de Watson for Oncology dans plus de soixante-dix centres médicaux réservés aux anciens combattants est censé venir en renfort des médecins, mais une future mise en service de l'IA en tant que clinicien de première ligne soulagerait le manque de main d'œuvre de façon plus immédiate. Grâce à cette solution, les patients de la VHA pourraient prendre rendez-vous en temps réel avec une IA pour des soins de base ou pour se voir prescrire une consultation chez un spécialiste, ce qui permettrait aux médecins en poste de répondre aux besoins des vétérans nécessitant des soins plus pointus.

En admettant que l'emploi de l'IA pour le diagnostic pourrait pourvoir aux besoins avérés de la VHA, il reste la deuxième condition nécessaire à l'utilisation éthique de cet outil technologique. Pour une utilisation éthique, les membres des forces armées américaines doivent pouvoir maintenir la relation médecin-patient dans le cadre de ce recours à l'IA en tant que

---

70. *The Use of Artificial Intelligence to Improve the U.S. Department of Veterans Affairs' Claims Processing System*, 2008. Hearing before the Subcommittee on Disability Assistance and Memorial Affairs of the Committee on Veterans' Affairs U.S. House of Representatives
71. Patricia Kime, "5 Years After Nationwide Scandal."

clinicien de première ligne. Fort heureusement, durant leur service, de nombreux militaires ont acquis une certaine capacité à forger des relations personnelles avec des outils technologiques d'avant-garde. C'est particulièrement évident au sein des unités de neutralisation, d'enlèvement et de destruction des engins explosifs (NEDEX) et dans leur emploi de robots démineurs, lequel a débuté en 1972.[72] Depuis le moment où ces engins ont été mis en service sur le terrain, les groupes d'intervention NEDEX ont démontré une capacité remarquable à tisser des liens émotionnels avec le robot démineur, au point où les unités lui donnaient un nom et le traitaient comme un animal de compagnie.[73] Certaines unités ont eu des liens suffisamment forts avec ces robots pour connaître un véritable sentiment de deuil et organiser des funérailles pour leur « compagnon d'arme » si le robot avait souffert des dommages irréparables[74]. Des exemples de groupes d'intervention NEDEX et de leurs robots tombés au champ d'honneur montrent que les soldats sont capables de forger des liens avec des entités non-humaines. De même, les anciens combattants atteints de troubles de stress post-traumatique (TSPT) ont montré un désir de divulguer plus de renseignements à un agent conversationnel intelligent qu'ils ne pourraient vouloir le faire dans une situation ordinaire.[75] Dans le stade actuel des choses, il semble que ces liens immédiats avec l'IA soient susceptibles de se développer vu la volonté avérée de l'armée de se tourner vers des technologies innovantes pour répondre aux besoins des militaires.

À travers l'histoire, la recherche militaire a été au premier plan des avancées médicales. Bien que le développement de ces technologies ait souvent des causes tragiques, l'armée a généralement constitué un environnement dans lequel les appareillages prothétiques ont connu de grandes avancées et les méthodes de sauvetage des membres et de leurs fonctions ont beaucoup progressé.[76] D'ailleurs, même les choses aussi basiques que les

---

72. Military.com, "The Very First Bomb Disposal Robot," January 15, 2014, https://www. military.com/video/ammunition-and-explosives/explosive-ordnance-disposal/the-first-bomb-disposal-robot/3059244734001.

73. Doree Armstrong, "Emotional Attachment to Robots Could Affect Outcome on Battlefield," Office of Minority Affairs Diversity, September 13, 2013, https://www. washington.edu/news/2013/09/17/emotional-attachment-to-robots-could-affect-outcome-on-battlefield/.

74. Megan Garber, "Funerals for Fallen Robots," *The Atlantic*. September 20, 2013. https:// www.theatlantic.com/technology/archive/2013/09/funerals-for-fallen-robots/279861/.

75. Myrthe L. Tielman et al., "A Therapy System for Post-Traumatic Stress Disorder."

76. Melissa Block, "Orthotic Brace Takes Soldiers from Limping to Leaping," *NPR*, March 31, 2014, https://www.npr.org/sections/health-shots/2014/03/31/295328707/orthotic-brace-takes-soldiers-from-limping-to-leaping.

garrots ou la production industrielle d'antibiotiques trouvent leurs sources dans le contexte militaire.[77] Ces avancées se sont ensuite étendues du contexte militaire à tous les systèmes de santé et on peut s'attendre à ce qu'il en soit de même pour les progrès médicaux à venir.

Une recherche déclassifiée en cours menée au sein de l'Agence pour les projets de recherche avancée de défense, la Defense Advanced Research Projects Agency (DARPA), fait mention d'un intérêt pour la mise en service de technologies médicales dotées d'IA au sein des armées. Un des programmes de la DARPA intitulé Warfighter Analytics using Smartphones for Health (WASH) entend mettre à profit la technologie présente dans les téléphones intelligents pour surveiller la santé et le niveau de préparation physique d'un soldat, comme une sorte de tracker de santé allant jusqu'à repérer des changements mineurs dans la démarche d'un soldat, dans sa tension musculaire et son niveau de transpiration.[78] Un autre projet annoncé pour 2019, Bioelectronics for Tissue Regeneration (BETR) axé sur la régénération tissulaire bioélectronique, entend associer l'IA à des capteurs pour suivre la réponse de l'organisme à des stimulations biochimiques ou biophysiques des tissus, le but étant de communiquer des données à des déclencheurs capables de cicatriser les blessures.[79] Alors que la technologie militaire avance et que l'IA s'intègre de plus en plus aux interactions humaines au sein de l'armée, les exemples de militaires qui développeront des liens avec la technologie durant leur carrière ne feront que se multiplier. Et en plus des interactions avec l'IA ayant lieu pendant leur carrière, les militaires des forces armées américaines auront également accès à la technologie intelligente destinée à la consommation de masse.

Ces interactions avec l'IA pourront établir les fondations sur lesquelles les militaires ayant besoin d'un traitement médical dans le cadre de la VHA pourront être soignés dans un délai convenable tout en maintenant le lien patient-médecin grâce à l'IA tenant le rôle du clinicien de première ligne. Évidemment, tous les militaires ne pourront avoir le même niveau d'interaction avec l'IA, en particulier les patients âgés qui n'avaient jamais été en contact avec l'IA durant leur carrière. Ainsi, de façon à adhérer

77. Leah Samuel, "6 Battlefield Medical Innovations That Moved to Mainstream Medicine," *STAT*, November 10, 2017, https://www.statnews.com/2017/11/10/medical-innovations-war/.

78. Jonathan M. Smith, "Warfighter Analytics Using Smartphones for Health (WASH)." https://www.darpa.mil/program/warfighter-analytics-using-smartphones-for-health.

79. Dr. Paul Sheehan, "Bioelectronics for Tissue Regeneration (BETR)." https://www.darpa.mil/program/bioelectronics-for-tissue-regeneration.

au plus près à un emploi éthique de l'IA pour le diagnostic, il devra être donné le choix aux militaires qui se feront soigner dans un centre médical réservé aux vétérans d'avoir affaire en premier lieu à une IA ou d'attendre qu'un médecin soit en mesure de les recevoir en consultation. À savoir qu'obliger un individu à faire ce choix en dépit de son confort, alors qu'il ne désire pas parler à un agent conversationnel ou profiter de l'assistance d'une IA pour effectuer le diagnostic d'un rhume ou d'une grippe, pourrait endommager le lien patient-médecin et rendre la mise en service de cette technologie bien peu éthique. Pourtant, étant donné la nature des progrès de la relation entre humanité et IA et les indications suggérant une future application dans les forces armées américaines, les années à venir verront probablement une augmentation du nombre des patients désireux d'interagir d'abord avec une IA. Comme nous l'avons évoqué précédemment, concernant les patients atteints de TSPT et leurs interactions avec un agent conversationnel et à propos du succès de la téléconsultation, il est possible que ces patients préfèrent s'en remettre à une IA, si cela implique qu'ils peuvent recevoir des soins immédiats.

Au cœur de la mise en service de l'IA se trouve un désir de dispenser de meilleurs soins qui soient plus ciblés et plus accessibles. Pour de nombreuses raisons, proposer l'application de l'IA en tant que clinicien de première ligne dans le système de santé américain constitue un grand défi dû à une méfiance sociétale bien ancrée envers l'IA. Toutefois, les préoccupations éthiques enracinées dans cette méfiance n'ont pas été suffisantes pour empêcher des avancées technologiques, et il est désormais impératif de réfléchir au-delà de l'hypothétique autorisation de l'emploi de l'IA en médecine pour orienter la conversation sur la question suivante : comment l'IA devrait-elle être mise en œuvre ? Dans le but d'assurer une utilisation éthique des futures technologies dans le système de santé, deux conditions doivent être remplies. À savoir que l'outil technologique doit servir un besoin documenté et que la mise en œuvre de la technologie ne doit pas endommager le potentiel d'évolution de la relation patient-médecin.

L'incapacité de la Veterans Health Administration à prendre pleinement en charge ses patients selon les standards établis pourrait être prise en compte à travers l'emploi de l'IA en tant que clinicien de première ligne. De surcroît, de nombreux membres des forces armées américaines qui à l'avenir seront pris en charge dans les centres médicaux réservés aux vétérans auront eu des interactions avec l'IA et forgé une relation unique avec les technologies de l'IA pendant leur carrière. Ces interactions pourraient donc les rendre capables de garder confiance en une décision médicale quand l'IA agit en tant que clinicien, et ce dans le respect du lien patient-clinicien. L'IA pourrait ne pas être encore tout à fait capable d'assumer pleinement ce rôle dans la phase du diagnostic, mais il est impératif d'anticiper une mise en œuvre éthique de l'IA dans l'avenir. Comme les futures technologies de l'IA amélioreront certainement les soins de santé, la Veterans Health Administration est susceptible de bénéficier considérablement de ces avancées, car elle constitue un environnement où la contribution de l'IA peut effectivement adhérer aux principes fondateurs de l'éthique médicale occidentale.

Références

American Hospital Association. "Fact Sheet: Telehealth." February 2019. https://www.aha.org/system/files/2019-02/fact-sheet-telehealth-2-4-19.pdf.

Ana, Cat. "Why the Japanese Find Deep Love with Deep Learning." *Medium. Becoming Human: Artificial Intelligence Magazine*, February 12, 2019. https://becominghuman.ai/why-the-japanese-find-deep-love-with-deep-learning-829e1bb629c2.

Armstrong, Doree. "Emotional Attachment to Robots Could Affect Outcome on Battlefield." Office of Minority Affairs Diversity. September 13, 2013. https://www.washington.edu/news/2013/09/17/emotional-attachment-to-robots-could-affect-outcome-on-battlefield/.

Asimov, Isaac. "Runaround" *I, Robot.* Greenwich, CT: Fawcett Publications, 1950.

Bickmore, Timothy W., Suzanne E. Mitchell, Brian W. Jack, Michael K. Paasche-Orlow, Laura M. Pfeifer, and Julie O'Donnell. "Response to a Relational Agent by Hospital Patients with Depressive Symptoms." *Interacting with Computers* 22, no. 4 (2010): 289–98.

Block, Melissa. "Orthotic Brace Takes Soldiers from Limping to Leaping." *NPR*, March 31, 2014. https://www.npr.org/sections/health-shots/2014/03/31/295328707/orthotic-brace-takes-soldiers-from-limping-to-leaping.

Bronstein, Scott, and Drew Griffin. "A Fatal Wait: Veterans Languish and Die on a VA Hospital's Secret List." *CNN*. Cable News Network, April 24, 2014. https://www.cnn.com/2014/04/23/health/veterans-dying-health-care-delays/index.html.

Builddie. "The Role of Artificial Intelligence in Wildlife Conservation." *Medium.* May 15, 2019. https://medium.com/builddie/the-role-of-artificial-intelligence-in-wildlife-conservation-5dc3af2b4222.

Business Wire. "Pacificor Names Latham & Watkins to Field Terminator Inquiries." Berkshire Hathaway. February 17, 2010. http://www.businesswire.com/news/home/20100217005514/en/Pacificor-Names-Latham-Watkins-Field-Terminator-Inquiries.

Eakins, Christopher, Wendy D. Ellis, Sumit Pruthi, David P. Johnson, Marta Hernanz-Schulman, Chang Yu, and J. Herman Kan. "Second Opinion Interpretations by Specialty Radiologists at a Pediatric Hospital: Rate of Disagreement and Clinical Implications." *American Journal of Roentgenology* 199, no. 4 (2012): 916–20.

Babylon Health, "Babylon AI Achieves Equivalent Accuracy with Human Doctors in Global Healthcare First." PR Newswire: News Distribution, Targeting and Monitoring. June 27, 2018. https://www.prnewswire.com/news-releases/babylon-ai-achieves-equivalent-accuracy-with-human-doctors-in-global-health-care-first-686718631.html.

Beauchamp, Thomas L., and James F. Childress. *Principles of Biomedical Ethics*. New York: Oxford University Press, 2013

Berner, Eta S. and Tonya J. La Lande, "Overview of Clinical Decision Support Systems," in *Clinical Decision Support Systems: Theory and Practice,* ed. Eta S. Berner. Switzerland: Springer International Press, 2016.

Bresnick, Jennifer. "Artificial Intelligence in Healthcare Market to See 40% CAGR Surge." HealthITAnalytics, July 24, 2017. https://healthitanalytics.com/news/artificial-intelligence-in-healthcare-market-to-see-40-cagr-surge.

Brown, Eric. "Watson: The *Jeopardy!* Challenge and beyond." 2013 IEEE 12th International Conference on Cognitive Informatics and Cognitive Computing, 2013.

Brynjolfsson, Erik, and Andrew McAfee. The Second Machine Age: Work, Progress, and Prosperity in a Time of Brilliant Technologies. Vancouver, BC: Langara College, 2018.

"Cleveland Clinic Express Care® Online." Cleveland Clinic. Accessed April 29, 2019. https://my.clevelandclinic.org/online-services/express-care-online.

Dyce, Andrew. "Our 10 Favorite Killer A.I.'s in Movies." Screen Rant, April 18, 2014. https://screenrant.com/artificial-intelligence-movies-evil-computers/.

Ehrenkranz, Melanie. "Facial Recognition Flags Woman on Bus Ad for 'Jaywalking' in China." *Gizmodo*. November 26, 2018. https://gizmodo.com/facial-recognition-flags-woman-on-bus-ad-for-jaywalking-1830654750.

Feldman, Robin C., Ehrik Aldana, and Kara Stein. 2019. "Artificial Intelligence in the Health Care Space: How can we trust what we cannot know." *Stanford Law & Policy Review* 30 (2): 399–419.

Garber, Megan. "Funerals for Fallen Robots." *The Atlantic.* September 20, 2013. https://www.theatlantic.com/technology/archive/2013/09/funerals-for-fallen-robots/279861/.

Hall, Mark A., Elizabeth Dugan, Beiyao Zheng, and Aneil K. Mishra. "Trust in Physicians and Medical Institutions: What Is It, Can It Be Measured, and Does It Matter?" *The Milbank Quarterly* 79, no. 4 (2001): 613–39.

Harmon, Amy. "A Soft Spot for Circuitry." *The New York Times*. July 5, 2010. https://www.nytimes.com/2010/07/05/science/05robot.html?_r=2&pagewanted=1.

Hosny, Ahmed, and Hugo J. W. L. Aerts. "Artificial Intelligence for Global Health." *American Association for the Advancement of Science*, November 22, 2019. https://science.sciencemag.org/content/366/6468/955.full.

Heckerman, David E., and Edward H. Shortliffe. "From Certainty Factors to Belief Networks." *Artificial Intelligence in Medicine* 4, no. 1 (1992): 35–52.

Iannitti, Tommaso, Alessandro Di Cerbo, Julio Cesar Morales-Medina, and Beniamino Palmieri. "Narrative Review of Telemedicine Consultation in Medical Practice." Patient Preference and Adherence, 2015, 65.

IBM. "Watson Overview." The DeepQA Research Team, July 25, 2016. https://researcher.watson.ibm.com/researcher/view_group.php?id=2099.

IBM Newsroom. "Manipal Hospitals Announces National Launch of IBM Watson for Oncology" IBM, July 26, 2016. https://www-03.ibm.com/press/in/en/pressrelease/50290.wss.

Ito, Joi. "Why Westerners Fear Robots and the Japanese Do Not." Wired. Conde Nast, July 30, 2018. https://www.wired.com/story/ideas-joi-ito-robot-overlords/.

Karches, Kyle E. 2018. "Against the IDoctor: Why Artificial Intelligence Should Not Replace Physician Judgment." *Theoretical Medicine and Bioethics* 39 (2): 91–110.

Kircher, Malone. "Yet Another Person Listens to GPS App and Drives Car Into Lake." *Intelligencer*, January 24, 2018. https://nymag.com/intelligencer/2018/01/waze-app-directs-driver-to-drive-car-into-lake-champlain.html.

Kime, Patricia. "5 Years After Nationwide Scandal, VA Still Struggles to Track Wait Times." Military.com, July 26, 2019. https://www.military.com/daily-news/2019/07/26/5-years-after-nationwide-scandal-va-still-struggles-track-wait-times.html.

Krupinski, Elizabeth A., Kevin S. Berbaum, Robert T. Caldwell, Kevin M. Schartz, and John Kim. "Long Radiology Workdays Reduce Detection and Accommodation Accuracy." *Journal of the American College of Radiology* 7, no. 9 (2010): 698–704.

Larin, Kathy. "Veterans health administration: Greater focus on credentialing needed to prevent disqualified providers from delivering patient care." Nova Science Publishers, Inc. 2019: 205-284.

Lee, Don. "Desperate for Workers, Aging Japan Turns to Robots for Healthcare." *Los Angeles Times*. July 25, 2019. https://www.latimes.com/world-nation/story/2019-07-25/desperate-for-workers-aging-japan-turns-to-robots-for-healthcare.

Matchar, Emily. "AI Plant and Animal Identification Helps Us All Be Citizen Scientists." Smithsonian.com. Smithsonian Institution, June 7, 2017. https://www.smithsonianmag.com/innovation/ai-plant-and-animal-identification-helps-us-all-be-citizen-scientists-180963525/.

Mather, Mark, Paola Scommegna, and Lillian Kilduff. "Fact Sheet: Aging in the United States." Population Reference Bureau, July 15, 2019. https://www.prb.org/aging-unitedstates-fact-sheet/

McGarry, Brendan. "VA Audit Confirms Veterans' Wait Times Complaints." Military.com, 2014. https://www.military.com/daily-news/2014/06/10/va-audit-confirms-veterans-wait-times-complaints.html.

Military.com. "The Very First Bomb Disposal Robot." January 15, 2014. https://www.military.com/video/ammunition-and-explosives/explosive-ordnance-disposal/the-first-bomb-disposal-robot/3059244734001.

National Science and Technology Council. "Emerging Technologies to Support an Aging Population." March 2019. https://www.whitehouse.gov/wp-content/uploads/2019/03/Emerging-Tech-to-Support-Aging-2019.pdf.

Oxford English Dictionary Online. "Artificial Intelligence." November 2019. Oxford: Oxford University Press. https://www.oed.com/view/Entry/271625?redirectedFrom=artificial+intelligence#eid.

Philipps, Dave. "Veterans Claiming Disability Pay Face Wall of Denials and Delays." *The New York Times*. November 13, 2017. https://www.nytimes.com/2017/11/13/us/veterans-affairs-department-benefits-delays.html.

Polakovic, Gary. "The next Big Effort in AI: Keeping L.A.'s Water Flowing Post-Earthquake." USC News, October 4, 2019. https://news.usc.edu/160680/ai-la-water-supply-earthquake-usc-research/.

Ross, Casey, and Ike Swetlitz. "IBM's Watson supercomputer recommended 'unsafe and incorrect' cancer treatments, internal documents show." STAT, July 25, 2018. https://www.statnews.com/2018/07/25/ibm-watson-recommended-unsafe-incorrect-treatments/.

Rosen, Dennis. *Vital Conversations: Improving Communication Between Doctors and Patients.* New York: Columbia University Press, 2014.

Russell, Stuart J., and Peter Norvig. *Artificial Intelligence a Modern Approach.* Boston: Pearson, 2016.

Samuel, Leah. "6 Battlefield Medical Innovations That Moved to Mainstream Medicine." STAT, November 10, 2017. https://www.statnews.com/2017/11/10/medical-innovations-war/.

Si, Ma, and Cheng Yu. "Chinese Robot Becomes World's First Machine to Pass Medical Exam." November 10, 2017. http://www.chinadaily.com.cn/bizchina/tech/2017-11/10/content_34362656.htm.

Sheehan, Dr. Paul. "Bioelectronics for Tissue Regeneration (BETR)." https://www.darpa.mil/program/bioelectronics-for-tissue-regeneration.

Smith, Jonathan M. "Warfighter Analytics Using Smartphones for Health (WASH)." https://www.darpa.mil/program/warfighter-analytics-using-smartphones-for-health.

Spitzer, Julie. "IBM's Watson recommended 'unsafe and incorrect' cancer treatments, STAT report finds." *Becker's Healthcare*, July 25, 2018. https://www.beckershospitalreview.com/artificial-intelligence/ibm-s-watson-recommended-unsafe-and-incorrect-cancer-treatments-stat-report-finds.html.

Strickland, Eliza. "How IBM Watson Overpromised and Underdelivered on AI Health Care." IEEE Spectrum: Technology, Engineering, and Science News. April 2, 2019. https://spectrum.ieee.org/biomedical/diagnostics/how-ibm-watson-overpromised-and-underdelivered-on-ai-health-care.

Tajitsu, Naomi. "Japanese Automakers Look to Robots to Aid the Elderly." *Scientific American.* April 12, 2017. https://www.scientificamerican.com/article/japanese-automakers-look-to-robots-to-aid-the-elderly/.

Tielman, Myrthe L., Mark A. Neerincx, Rafael Bidarra, Ben Kybartas, and Willem-Paul Brinkman. "A Therapy System for Post-Traumatic Stress Disorder Using a Virtual Agent and Virtual Storytelling to Reconstruct Traumatic Memories." Journal of Medical Systems 41, no. 8 (2017): 125.

Truschel, Jessica. "Top 25 Mental Health Apps for 2020: An Alternative to Therapy?" Psycom.net–Mental Health Treatment Resource Since 1986, March 19, 2020. https://www.psycom.net/25-best-mental-health-apps.

United States Bureau of Labor Statistics. "Home Health Aides and Personal Care Aides: Occupational Outlook Handbook," September 4, 2019. https://www.bls.gov/ooh/healthcare/home-health-aides-and-personal-care-aides.htm.

Vaidyam, Aditya, and John Torous. "Chatbots: What Are They and Why Care?" *Psychiatric Times*. June 27, 2019. https://www.psychiatrictimes.com/telepsychiatry/chatbots-what-are-they-and-why-care.

Vincent, James. "Twitter Taught Microsoft's Friendly AI Chatbot to Be a Racist Asshole in Less Than a Day." *The Verge*. March 24, 2016. https://www.theverge.com/2016/3/24/11297050/tay-microsoft-chatbot-racist.

Vincent, James. "Google's AI Thinks This Turtle Looks like a Gun, Which Is a Problem." *The Verge*. November 2, 2017. https://www.theverge.com/2017/11/2/16597276/google-ai-image-attacks-adversarial-turtle-rifle-3d-printed.

Yan, Alice. "How a Robot Passed China's Medical Licensing Exam." *South China Morning Post*, November 20, 2017. Accessed April 20, 2019.

Yu, V. L. "Antimicrobial Selection by a Computer. A Blinded Evaluation by Infectious Diseases Experts." *JAMA: The Journal of the American Medical Association* 242, no. 12 (1979): 1279–282.

Contributors and Translators

Sara Gaines earned her MA in Bioethics and Medical Humanities at the Case Western Reserve University. She is now pursuing a PhD in History at CWRU, focusing on the history of artificial intelligence.

Laura Graham earned her PhD at University of Aberdeen, Scotland and her JD at Case Western Reserve University. She is currently an Honors Attorney at the US Department of Justice in Washington, DC.

Nathan Riehl earned his MA in Philosophy at the University of Pennsylvania. He is currently an Instructor at the United States Military Academy, West Point, and a major in the United States Army.

French Translations
Fabienne Pizot-Haymore, translator
Nathalie Letourneau, proofreader

Spanish Translators
Haydeé Espino, translator
Victoria A. García, proofreader